NARCOTICS AND CELL NARCOSIS IN CHEMOTHERAPY

by

V. P. Paribok

Authorized translation from the Russian

Springer Science+Business Media, LLC 1962

The Russian text was published by
the USSR Academy of Sciences Press,
in Moscow and Leningrad in 1961

Всеволод Петрович Парибок
НАРКОТИКИ И КЛЕТОЧНЫЙ НАРКОЗ В ХИМИОТЕРАПИИ
NARKOTIKI I KLETOCHNYI NARKOZ V KHIMIOTERAPII

Library of Congress Catalog Card Number 62-12855

ISBN 978-1-4899-4895-3   ISBN 978-1-4899-4893-9 (eBook)
DOI 10.1007/978-1-4899-4893-9

© 1962 Springer Science+Business Media New York
Originally published by Consultants Bureau Enterprises, Inc. in 1962.

CONTENTS

PREFACE

Chemotherapy deals with the specific treatment of infectious diseases by means of chemical substances, and it dates from the late nineteenth and early twentieth centuries. The guiding principle of chemotherapy is selective toxicity, the selective poisoning of the agent of the disease by the drug with the minimal injury to the host (the patient or sick animal). It is supposed that only those substances which bear a special relationship to the pathogenic agent, initially defined as an "affinity" or "tropism," may have a selective action on it. This principle was formulated by Paul Ehrlich (1907) as follows: "I aimed at specific therapy, i.e., I sought chemical substances which, on the one hand, would be taken up by particular parasites and be capable of killing them, and on the other hand, would be tolerated by the host without great harm in the doses required to kill the parasites. If we call...substances fixed by the parasite 'etiotropic' and those fixed by the host 'organotropic,' the therapeutic application of such specific drugs will be rational only if their etiotropy is much stronger than their organotropy" (Ehrlich, 1907, p. 85).

Advances in the biochemistry of microorganisms led to the elucidation of the indefinite concept of "affinity" as the ability of a drug to compete with factors from the environment essential to the microorganisms, by virtue of the similarity of its chemical structure (Woolley, 1954). The harmlessness or low toxicity of chemotherapeutic agents is due to differences between the metabolic processes of the parasites and host.

Modern chemotherapy possesses the means to act upon the agents causing many infectious and parasitic diseases: on bacteria, viruses, protozoa, and also on multicellular organisms such as helminths. Chemotherapeutic agents are much older than the science of chemotherapy; the oldest of them are the anthelminthics. The expulsion of intestinal helminths is amenable to direct observation, so that a very clear criterion of the efficacy of anthelminthic drugs is available. Some current anthelminthics were chosen from among natural compounds some two thousand years ago, i.e., long before anything was known of the causes and ways of spread of the helminthiases. It is interesting to note that more recent researches have not led to the supplanting of these drugs; some of them even today are counted among the most effective (santonin, the active principle of Artemisia maritima, preparations of male fern, and so on).

The chemotherapy of the helminthiases, initially empirical, subsequently recognized and now uses the principle of selective toxicity to explain the lethal action of the drugs on the parasite. This principle is the only one which is possible in the treatment of helminthiases, the agents of which inhabit the organs and tissues outside the intestine. So far as the treatment of the intestinal helminthiases and of some helminthiases of the liver is concerned, in these cases the principle of selective toxicity may be supplemented by the use of the principle of selective accumulation of the chemotherapeutic agents in the habitat of the parasites. This principle is as follows.

Besides substances which are selectively toxic to the parasites, other substances may have a therapeutic action, even if they are less toxic to the parasite than to the host, provided that for some reason or other they can accumulate at the place where the parasites are to be found. It is obvious that this type of chemotherapeutic action can be used only under the following conditions: the ability of the substances to accumulate at the habitat of the parasite, which is measured by the ratio between the concentration at this place and the concentration in the blood, must be higher than the ratio between the toxicity of the substance to the host and to the parasite. In other words, the lower toxicity of the drug to the parasite must be "canceled out" by its selective accumulation at the habitat of the parasite.

At first glance this case appears extremely unpromising. In fact, the main trend in chemotherapeutic research is to look for a substance which is more toxic to the parasite than to the host to the greatest possible degree. Nevertheless, substances whose action is based on the principle of selective accumulation are also very widely used in chemotherapy (see Chapter 1).

The properties postulated above of chemotherapeutic agents acting in accordance with the principle of selective accumulation are shown in the clearest manner by the narcotics. Narcotics have the ability to depress temporarily the vital activity of a great variety of organisms, from unicellular to the higher animals. As shown by work done in D. N. Nasonov's laboratory (Makarov, 1938), animals may be divided into two types in accordance with the mechanism of narcosis and, correspondingly, with their sensitivity to narcotics: highly sensitive species, in which narcosis is a reversible depression of the function of the nervous system, and species of low sensitivity, in which narcosis is accompanied by depression of the vital activity of all the somatic cells. In the first case we speak of narcosis of nervous type, and in the second case, of narcosis of cellular type.

Vertebrate animals, the hosts of helminths, exhibit narcosis of nervous type. They are more sensitive to narcotics than are helminths. In contrast, narcosis in helminths is of the cellular type. Narcosis is of the same type in the parasitic protozoa.

Narcotics are less toxic to protozoa and helminths than to mammals, but they are capable of accumulating temporarily in certain habitats of the parasites in a higher concentration than in the organism as a whole. Because of this fact, they have a toxic action on the parasites.

The chemotherapeutic effect of narcotics must be regarded as a manifestation of cellular narcosis in chemotherapy. The object of this book is to establish the grounds for this statement and to use it in the search for new chemotherapeutic agents.

Chapter 1

NARCOTICS IN THE CHEMOTHERAPY OF THE HELMINTHIASES

1. The Use of Narcotics in the Chemotherapy of Helminthic Infestation

Chlorine-substituted hydrocarbons. In the second half of the nineteenth century, when surgical anesthesia gained fame and became widely practiced, many attempts were made to extend the scope of medical application of narcotics and to use them for other purposes than anesthesia. One such attempt was reported by Bennet (1885), who used chloroform to treat infestation with tapeworms, with good results.

Reports of the use of chloroform for a similar purpose were subsequently made by Hall (1919), Cawston (1945) and Le Dentu (1949). Because of the inadequacy of its therapeutic power, chloroform never achieved popularity as an anthelminthic drug. Guided by the idea of chemical analogy, Hall (1921) suggested that not only chloroform, but also other chlorine-substituted hydrocarbons, may have an anthelminthic action. He tested carbon tetrachloride in cases of ankylostomiasis; the drug was highly effective and quickly achieved popularity. It began to be used with varying success in other helminthic infestations than ankylostomiasis, in both medical and veterinary practice: in enterobiasis (Tuaev, 1936, 1954), in trematodiases of farm animals (Il'inskii and Palimpsestov, 1929; El'manov,1929; Shul'ts and Sutyagin, 1934), in nematodiases of domestic birds (Pukhov, 1932), and in many other helminthiases (see the survey in the book by Shul'ts, 1931).

Besides the generally positive evaluation of this new anthelminthic drug, some adverse comments were also published: it was reported that carbon tetrachloride may cause serious poisoning of the liver and kidneys. This led to a search for equally effective but less toxic anthelminthic drugs. Because the anthelminthic action of two chlorinated hydrocarbons ($CHCl_3$ and CCl_4) was already known, tests of the haloid-substituted hydrocarbons were continued.

Hall and Shillinger (1925) reported that tetrachlorotheylene ($CCl_2 = CCl_2$) was highly effective in ankylostomiasis and ascariasis in dogs. Tetrachlorotheylene was just as effective as carbon tetrachloride, but much less toxic to higher animals. Not a single fatality was reported during the treatment of human patients with tetrachloroethylene, whereas the use of carbon tetrachloride, for example, in Egypt caused the death of seven or eight persons each year as a result of the side effects of the drug. Tetrachloroethylene does not injure the liver of the other parenchymatous organs.

Just like carbon tetrachloride, tetrachloroethylene acts not only on hookworms, but also on other species of helminths, for example, on Ascaris and Trichuris (Hall and Augustine, 1929), although it is less effective in ascariasis (Kamalov and Tavlalishvili, 1951). In veterinary practice, tetrachloroethylene is used mainly in ascariasis and the ankylostomiasis of domestic animals and game (Machul'skii, 1938, 1941; Petrov et al., 1935; Sutyagin, 1941). It is ineffective against trematodes, which are parasites of the biliary passages (Shul'ts and Davtyan, 1934).

Besides carbon tetrachloride and tetrachloroethylene, one more preparation belonging to the group of chlorinated hydrocarbons has been introduced into medical and veterinary practice: hexachloroethane (CCl_3—CCl_3). This has proved most effective in fascioliasis: infestation of the biliary passages by the liver fluke. Hexachloroethane was originally used as a component of the proprietary preparation "neoserapis"; it was soon found, however, that the only active substance in this composite preparation is hexachloroethane. Subsequently, hexachloroethane began to be used in the pure form (Davtyan, 1937, 1940; Potemkina, 1945; Perikhanyan and Zorabyan, 1948; and others).

The efficacy of hexachloroethane in another liver infestation, opisthorchiasis, was first discovered by Plotnikov (1941) and studied in greater detail by his colleague Kovalev (1953). Kovalev tested several drugs on dogs with fistula of the common bile duct, infested with the trematode Opisthorchis felineus. In this type of experiment the trematodes expelled by the action of the anthelminthic drugs did not enter the intestine, but were passed externally and could easily be detected and counted.

Wright and co-workers (1932, 1937) made a systematic investigation of the anthelminthic action of many haloid-substituted hydrocarbons in experiments on animals; many of these compounds were effective. Their anthelminthic action did not exhibit narrow specificity, i.e., it was not confined to one species of helminths, helminths belonging to different families or even different orders (for example, nematodes and cestodes).

Carbohydrates. Petroleum, a natural mixture of hydrocarbons, was used for the treatment of worm infestations by oriental physicians during the Middle Ages (Éfendiev, 1947). Benzine (Hall and Foster, 1918) and kerosene (Faure, 1940; Baskakov et al., 1944; Velichkin and Khrapov, 1946, 1947; Kadenatsii, 1947; Selivanov, 1948) are very occasionally used in veterinary practice, mainly for lack of more effective anthelminthic substances. Benzine is also used occasionally in medical helminthology. Biyal (1948) treated ascariasis in human patients with purified benzine and obtained good results in 60 of 67 cases; in teniasis good results were obtained in 44 of 48 cases. Gieron (1954) treated patients suffering from ascariasis, trichocephaliasis, oxyuriasis or teniasis with benzine, and observed expulsion of the helminths in 47 of 52 patients. Benzine was reported to be highly effective in teniasis by Wigand and Warnecke (1953) and Niemirski (1954).

It must be pointed out that benzine and kerosene are not widely used as anthelminthic drugs. To obtain good results, it is necessary to give very large doses of the preparations. Biyal and Gieron, for example, gave their patients 60 ml (!) of benzine. This dosage made administration of the drug difficult, for both preparations possess unpleasant organoleptic properties. Another important feature is that benzine and kerosene are products of variable composition (Lazarev, 1954), and the efficacy of different samples may accordingly vary considerably.

The anthelminthic action of the hydrocarbons hexane and cyclohexane was first observed by Whitlock (1945), but these drugs did not prove highly effective. An anthelminthic action is characteristic not only of the aliphatic and cyclic hydrocarbons, but also of aromatic compounds such as toluene (Blair, 1949; Enzie, 1947; Enzie and Colglasier, 1953; Todd and Brown, 1952).

Of the total number of anthelminthic compounds mentioned in this chapter, only one — chloroform — is used as an anesthetic in surgery. The rest, although not surgical anesthetics, are nevertheless narcotics in the pharmacological sense (see, for example, the survey by Lazarev, 1940). The narcotic action of these substances on the host bears no relation to their efficacy as anthelminthics. Their anthelminthic action is exhibited in the absence or, in the most unfavorable cases, in the presence of only the initial signs of depression of the central nervous system of the host. The compound having the most marked side effects, namely chloroform, is also the least effective of the narcotics in its anthelminthic action.

Do these substances act as narcotics on helminths? This suggestion was first made by Lazarev (1944a, 1944b). On the subject of the anthelminthic action of carbon tetrachloride, tetrachloroethylene and similar compounds, he wrote: "A further question is whether special effects of these compounds are significant here; whether, on the other hand, they are simply narcotics in relation to the parasite, and are only slowly absorbed by the host and, at the same time, are rapidly excreted through the lungs. The whole affair probably rests on suitable combinations of the Overton—Meyer coefficient of these substances (indicating the strength of their narcotic action), their absolute solubility in water (an important factor in the rate of solution in the intestine and in the rate of absorption), and sometimes, perhaps, their coefficient of distribution between blood and air (the rate of elimination through the lungs of the compound absorbed by the host). These considerations lead to the thought that among the organic fluids of groups V-VII* an attempt may be made to select substances with an identical or even enhanced vermifugal effect by a suitable combination of their physicochemical properties" (Lazarev, 1944b, p. 189).

Later in this chapter we shall give information which may be regarded as indirect evidence in support of this hypothesis. This includes: the broad spectrum of anthelminthic action of the narcotics, the external pattern of their action on helminths (in particular, the reversibility of the effect), and the correlation between their physicochemical properties and their anthelminthic action.

2. The Spectrum of the Chemotherapeutic Action of Anthelminthic Narcotics

We have previously mentioned that anthelminthics of the carbon tetrachloride type in contrast, for example, to santonin are used in the treatment of infestations by a great variety of helminths, far removed from each other in a systematic respect. Carbon tetrachloride was introduced into helminthological practice as a drug for the treatment of ankylostomiasis. It was subsequently discovered that this compound was effective in enterobiasis (Tuaev, 1954), and that it acts on tapeworms (Maplestone and Mukerji, 1931; Pod'yapol'skaya, 1945; Zenaishvili, 1951), and also on trematodes (Plotnikov and Zerchaninov, 1932).

---

*This refers to the classification of nonelectrolytes suggested by Lazarev (1944a, 1944b).

TABLE 1. The Action of Anthelminthic Drugs on Cestodes and Nematodes (Rebello et al., 1928)

Substance	Cestodes Taenia serrata, Dipylidium caninum	Nematodes	
		Ascaris suum	Anklyostoma brasiliense
Infusion of kuosso	++++	0	0
Kamala (infusion)	++++	0	0
Infusion of fern	++++	0	0
Ethereal extract of fern	++++	0	0
Filmaron	++++	0	0
Decoction of pomegranate bark	++	0	0
Pelletierin	++	0	0
Pseudopelletierin	0	0	0
Arecoline	+	+	++
Oil of chenopodium	++++	++++	++
Thymol	++++	++++	++++
Betanaphthol	++++	++++	++++
Carbon tetrachloride	++++	++	++++
Santonin	+	+++	++
Allyl sulfide	+	+++	0
Pyridine	0	++++	+
Nicotine	0	++++	±

Note: "0" denotes no effect; the greater the number of plus signs, the stronger the action; the sign ± denotes a doubtful effect.

Thymol, which may also be classed as an anthelminthic drug of this type (the proof of this statement will be given later), was originally introduced for the treatment of ankylostomiasis, but was subsequently used for other infestations: for trichocephaliasis, enterobiasis, teniasis, and trematodiasis (Pod'yapol'skaya and Kapustin, 1958).

Admittedly, a given drug is not equally effective in the treatment of different helminthiases. However, this may depend not only on true differences in the sensitivity of the helminths to the action of the preparation, but also on several other causes, notably, for example, on the different localization of the various species of helminths in the gastrointestinal tract. When the sensitivity of the different helminths to a given drug is being compared, it is therefore important to use the results of experiments performed in vitro rather than in vivo, i.e., experiments on helminths outside the body of the host. Many such investigations have been carried out. The results of one of these are shown in Table 1. The activity of various anthelminthic drugs tested by Rebello and co-workers (1928) in experiments on nematodes and cestodes is expressed in conventional units and denoted by plus signs. It will be clear from Table 1 that besides the anthelminthic drugs which act almost exclusively on cestodes or on nematodes, there are others which are equally toxic to both orders of helminths. These include oil of chenopodium, thymol betanaphthol, and carbon tetrachloride.

There is thus no doubt that one drug may be used to act upon members of different classes and even orders of parasitic helminths. The ability to exert a toxic action on members of different systematic groups of the animal world is a characteristic feature of the narcotics. The polytropic anthelminthic action of carbon tetrachloride and other compounds is therefore of great importance as evidence of the narcotic nature of their action.

3. The Action of Anthelminthic Drugs on the Motor Activity of Helminths

Helminths extracted from the bowel can survive for some time in artificial media and maintain their motor activity. The influence of anthelminthic drugs on the movement of helminths in these conditions has been the subject of many experimental investigations. Rebello and co-workers (1928) tested carbon tetrachloride, among other substances. This compound caused immobility of nematodes (Ascaris and Ankylostoma) and also of the cestodes Taenia serrata and Dipylidium caninum. The fact that the paralytic action of carbon tetrachloride on the cestode Moniezia expansa is reversible by washing off the drug was described by Duguid and Heathcote (1950). Oelkers and Rathye (1941) observed reversible depression of the movements of ascarides after the action of chloroform, carbon

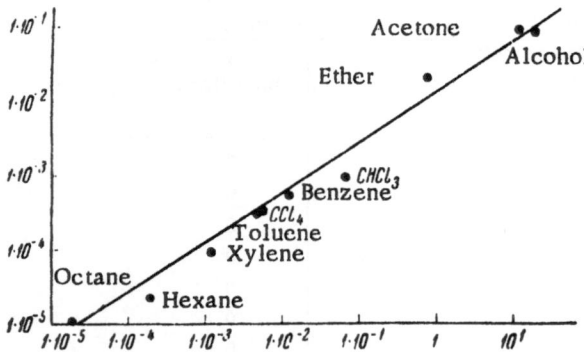

Fig. 1. Relationship between the strength of the narcotic action of nonelectrolytes and their solubility in water. Along the axis of abscissas — solubility in water (moles/ liter); along the axis of ordinates — narcotic concentration in mammalian blood (in true aqueous solution, in moles/ liter). Logarithmic scale. Plotted from figures cited by Lazarev (1944b, 1954).

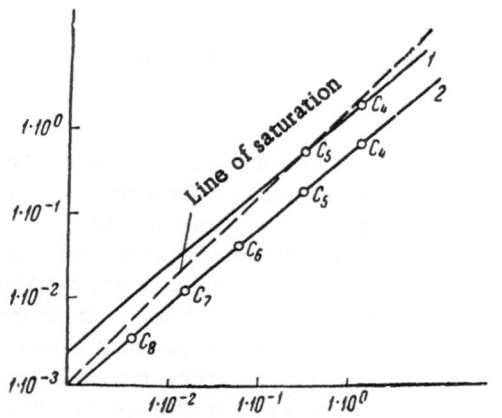

Fig. 2. Relationship between the solubility in water and the bactericidal action of alcohols on Staphylococcus aureus (1) and Eberthella typh- osa (2). Along the axis of abscissas — solubility in water (moles/ liter); along the axis of ordi- nates — toxic concentration (moles/ liter). C_4-C_8: alcohols from butyl to octyl. Data from Albert (1953).

tetrachloride, and tetrachloroethylene. When the helminths were transferred to a medium free from the narcotic, their movements were restored. These workers obtained similar results with nonparasitic worms (enchitreides). Depression of the movements of ascarides by carbon tetrachloride was found by Krotov (1953).

A noteworthy feature of these investigations is the reversibility of the depression of the movements of the helminths as a result of the action of anthelminthic narcotic drugs. In other cases (the action of fern preparations, santonin, or oxygen) reversibility is either absent or only partial. It will be remembered that reversibility of the effect is a characteristic feature of the action of narcotics.

4. The Relationship Between the Physicochemical Properties and the Action of Anthelminthic Drugs

The narcotic action extends to very widely different organisms: from protozoa to the higher animals and man. The ability of narcotics to cause reversible (within certain limits) depression of reactions is a special case of the biological action of nonelectrolytes. The principles governing the relationship between the biological action of nonelectrolytes and their physicochemical properties are the same for different biological effects: narcotic, hemolytic, lethal, bactericidal, etc.

We accordingly speak of nonelectrolytic action (Lazarev) — the pharmacological action of nonelectrolytes, closely associated with their physicochemical properties and not depending on chemical reactions or on conversion of active substances. The fact that the nonelectrolytic action is independent of chemical reactions in which nonelectrolytes may take part is proved conclusively by the narcotic action of the inert gases, which cannot take part in any reaction (Lazarev, 1941; Lazarev, Lyublina and Madorskaya, 1948; Lawrence et al., 1946).

The justification for combining the various effects characterizing the nonelectrolytes into the general concept of nonelectrolytic action is no less evident than that for distinguishing, for example, electrolytic or ionic effects, the common feature of which is the participation of electrically charged particles — ions — in the reaction.

Nonelectrolytic action may be contrasted with specific, based on a chemical reaction between the poison and the protoplasm. Under these circumstances, the specific action of a given poison does not exclude the possibility of a nonelectrolytic action, which may develop in this case when the concentration of the drug is increased.

In a series of nonelectrolytes the intensity of the biological (for example, narcotic) action of the compounds changes in accordance with their physicochemical properties. There is a particularly clear relationship between the biological action of nonelectrolytes and their properties of adhesion (Lazarev, 1940, 1944), i.e., with the properties of the substances determined by the magnitude of their adhesion to (affinity for) water, their solubility, surface activity, and so on. One example of such a relationship is shown in Fig. 1. The narcotic concentrations of certain nonelectrolytes vary in very close correlation with their solubility in water. As the solubility in water decreases, the narcotic action becomes stronger. Similar results may be obtained by comparing different forms of nonelectrolytic action with other adhesion properties, for example, with the magnitude of the Overton—Meyer coefficient, which

TABLE 2. Treatment of Ankylostomiasis in Dogs by Bromine-Substituted Hydrocarbons (Wright, Schaffer, Bozicevich, and Underwood, 1937)

Substance	Solubility in water	% of helminths removed from the bowel as a result of treatment
Propyl bromide	1:400	58.1
Butyl bromide	1:1600	99.2
Amyl bromide	1:6000	84
Hexyl bromide	1:12000	48.3
Heptyl bromide	1:30000	33

describes quantitatively the distribution of the substance between two immiscible phases, with the magnitude of their surface action, and so on.

The close connection between the physicochemical properties of narcotics and their biological action is evidence of the physicochemical nature of the action of narcotics and of the fact that the narcotic effect is independent of the ability of the molecules to take part in chemical reactions. Hence it follows that the data relating to the relationship between the physicochemical properties and the action of anthelminthic drugs, which we shall examine in this section, are of great importance to the explanation of the mechanism of their anthelminthic action.

TABLE 3. The Ascaricidal Action of Alkyl Metacresols (Lamson and Brown, 1935c)

Substance	Solubility in water	Duration of action								
		in minutes						in hours		
		2	3	10	20	30	45	1	2	3
m-Cresol	1:40	0	0	0	0	0	0	0	0	0
6-Methyl-m-cresol	1:450	0	0	0	0	0	0	0	0	0
6-Ethyl-m-cresol	1:750	0	0	0	0	0	0	50	100	100
6-n-Propyl-m-cresol	1:4000	20	60	90	100	100	100	100	100	100
6-n-Butyl-m-cresol	1:6000	14	100	100	100	100	100	100	100	100
6-n-Amyl-m-cresol	1:50,000	9	12	100	100	100	100	100	100	100
6-n-Hexyl-m-cresol	1:150,000	4	9	52	60	98	100	100	100	100
6-n-Heptyl-m-cresol	1:600,000	0	20	58	67	92	100	100	100	100
6-n-Octyl-m-cresol	-	0	0	50	50	50	50	50	100	100
6-n-Nonyl-m-cresol	-	0	0	0	12	12	25	50	50	75

Note. The figures in the table correspond to the proportion of immobilized ascarides in percent.

When the physicochemical properties and the action of anthelminthic drugs have been compared, the greatest attention has been paid to their solubility in water. We drew attention above to only one aspect of the pattern of the relationship between the action of narcotics and their solubility in water: the increase in strength of the effect of a series of narcotics in order of decreasing solubility. Another aspect is the limiting role of solubility. The strengthening of the narcotic action during the transition to less soluble narcotics has an upper limit. When the solubility is slight, it is insufficient to exhibit a biological effect, so that in a series of narcotics arranged in descending order of solubility, the increase in effect is replaced by its disappearance. For example, in a series of alcohols, all tested homologs have an action on Eberthella typhosa (Fig. 2); only butyl and amyl alcohols act on Staphylococcus aureus, for the higher alcohols are insufficiently soluble. The reason for this is as follows. In a series of nonelectrolytes (for example, in a homologous series) the solubility of the compounds in water changes during the transition from the lower members of the series to the higher in accordance with a quantitatively different law from that obeyed by the biological action. The decrease in solubility is more rapid than the increase in toxicity of the nonelectrolytes. This principle was discovered independently by Ferguson (1939) and Lazarev (1944b). Lazarev showed that the same assertion is justified when the action of substances from different homologous series is being compared.

For this reason an optimal solubility must exist (and is, in fact, observed) in respect to the different forms of biological action of the nonelectrolytes: readily soluble substances have a weak action, and insoluble substances do not act at all; the most active substances are those whose solubility in water occupies some intermediate position. This phenomenon may also be found when the anthelminthic action of narcotics is compared with their solubility.

Wright and Schaffer (1932) compared the anthelminthic action of many chlorinated hydrocarbons in dogs with ascariasis and ankylostomiasis. They found that, whereas the solubility of substances in a homologous series decreases regularly and continuously from the lower homologs to the higher, their efficacy reaches a definite maximum and then falls. These writers concluded that the efficacy of the chlorinated hydrocarbons is largely determined by their solubility in water. In ankylostomiasis the most effective substances have a solubility from 1:1250 to 1:5300, and in ascariasis from 1:350 to 1:3500. Another example illustrating this principle can be found in the work of Wright et al. (1937). Bromine-substituted hydrocarbons, like the chlorine-substituted compounds, have an anthelminthic action. In ankylostomiasis in dogs, in a series of these compounds the efficacy reaches a maximum with butyl bromide (Table 2).

Shul'ts (1933) emphasizes the presence of an optimum of solubility, associated with maximal anthelminthic action, in the series:

$$C_2Cl_6 < C_2Cl_4 > CCl_4 > CHCl_3$$

greater $\longleftarrow$ solubility $\longrightarrow$ less

The solubility decreases from left to right, whereas the anthelminthic action reaches its maximum with tetra-chloroethylene.

In a series of investigations, Lamson, Brown, and others (1935a, 1935b, 1935c, 1935d, 1935e) studied the action of numerous alkylhydroxybenzenes on ascarides. These compounds were synthesized because of the need to find a more effective and less toxic anthelminthic substance than hexylresorcinol (Lamson et al., 1930). Figures showing the relationship between the solubility of alkyl metacresols and their ascaricidal action, obtained in one of these investigations, are given in Table 3.

The maximum of efficacy is very clearly seen in the substances having a solubility between 1:4000 and 1:6000. The same conclusions may be drawn from the results of other investigations of this series conducted by Lamson and his co-workers.

Investigations of the anthelminthic efficacy of haloid-substituted hydrocarbons and alkylhydroxybenzenes thus reveal very similar phenomena. In both cases there is a maximum of efficacy at a definite optimum of solubility of the compounds in water. This fact supports the hypothesis that their anthelminthic action is narcotic in nature, for similar correlations between solubility and toxicity are also characteristic of other forms of narcotic (nonelectrolytic) action.

Neither this fact, nor the width of the spectrum of anthelminthic action of the narcotics, nor the reversibility of the depression of movement of the helminths in their solution, is direct evidence of the nonelectrolytic mechanism of their action. Width of their chemotherapeutic spectrum is characteristic, for example, of certain antibiotics: chlortetracycline, tetracycline, and others, the mechanism of whose antibacterial action is in no way nonelectrolytic in nature. Moreover, reversibility of the injury within certain limits is also characteristic of the action not only of narcotics, but also of other physical and chemical factors of the environment. The association between the biological action and the physicochemical properties of poisons is also found in cases of frankly specific types of action, and it is by no means confined to nonelectrolytic effects.

Meanwhile, these principles, each of which is not confined in its application to narcotic action alone, when taken together make it more likely that the mechanism of the anthelminthic action of carbon tetrachloride, tetra-chloroethylene, and similar compounds is one of narcosis.

Chapter 2

THE NONELECTROLYTIC ACTION OF ANTHELMINTHIC DRUGS

1. Narcosis of Helminths — Narcosis of the Cellular Type

In response to the action of very different stimuli, a group of nonspecific, uniform changes takes place in the protoplasm: the degree of dispersion of the colloids forming the cytoplasm and nucleus decreases, the viscosity of the cytoplasm increases and its power of fixing vital dyes is strengthened, certain substances are liberated and leave the cell while others, on the contrary, enter it from the surrounding medium where they are usually found. This group of changes, reversible in the initial stage, is called paranecrosis (Nasonov and Aleksandrov, 1940; Nasonov, 1959). Among the stimuli causing paranecrotic changes are the narcotics. Narcosis of the cell, as a functional phenomenon, arises when changes develop in the substance of the protoplasm, i.e., paranecrosis.

Narcosis of the lower animals arises only in response to relatively high concentrations of narcotics, the action of which leads to the development of paranecrotic changes in all the body cells. In contrast to this, narcosis arises in the higher animals, for example, mammals, in response to low concentrations of narcotics, insufficient to cause paranecrotic changes in the cells. The cell substance remains unchanged and functionally intact. Narcosis develops as a result of injury to the nervous system (Makarov, 1938).

Helminths and the animals in which they live (vertebrates) may belong to various types depending on their sensitivity to narcotics: a first or low-sensitive type and a second or highly-sensitive type. The narcotic concentrations of, for example, chloroform for vertebrates are of a lower order than those for helminths (Table 4). Hence, the following conclusion may be drawn: if carbon tetrachloride and certain other anthelminthic drugs act on helminths as narcotics, they must be less toxic toward them than toward the higher animals. In other words, in contrast to all the chemotherapeutic drugs — the sulfonamides, antibiotics, and so on — the organotropic property of these substances must be stronger than the etiotropic. One method of elucidating the mechanism of their action (narcotic or other specific action) must therefore be to compare their toxicity toward the host (a higher animal), on the one hand, and toward the helminths, on the other.

Many investigations have been carried out from which figures may be obtained in respect to the toxicity of anthelminthic drugs toward helminths: lethal or toxic concentrations. Some of these results will be described in this chapter.

So far as the toxicity of anthelminthic drugs toward the host (a higher animal) is concerned, no such information is available. Frequent determinations have been made of the therapeutic, toxic, and lethal doses of anthelminthic drugs for various species of animals, for enteral or parenteral administration. Some studies have been made of histological changes found in animals after administration of therapeutic or toxic doses. These figures cannot, however, be used to elucidate the problem with which we are concerned. The only adequate characteristic of the toxicity of a substance, both toward the helminth and toward the host, is the concentration at which the effects interesting the experimenter are found. In experiments on higher animals such an index is the blood concentration of the poison, for example, the lethal concentration. This may be compared with the concentration of the same poison exerting a toxic action on helminths , and the ratio between the toxicity of the substance toward helminths and toward their host may thereby be determined.

2. The Toxic Concentration of Anthelminthic Drugs in the Blood of Animals

In experiments on cats we determined the lethal concentrations of the following anthelminthic drugs: carbon tetrachloride, tetrachloroethylene, hexylresorcinol, and thymol, and the minimal toxic concentration of santonin. We also determined the toxicity of oxygen to cats, for it has been used with success in the treatment of ascariasis. Santonin and oxygen, the action of which on helminths may , for several considerations, be regarded as specific, were used for comparison with the remaining drugs.

TABLE 4. Narcotic Concentrations of Chloroform for Various Species of Animals (according to Makarov, 1938)

Order	Class	Species	Narcotic concentration, in millimoles
Protozoa	Infusoria	Balantidium	6
		Nyctotherus	12
		Vorticella microstomata	12
		Pyxidium sp.	12
	Flagellata	Opalina ranarum	12
Platyhelminthes	Cestoda	Dolychosaccus rastellus	12
		Haplometra cylindrocoelum	12
Nemathelminthes	Nematoda	Rhabditis sp.	12
Arthropoda	Arachnoidea	—	1.5
	Insecta	Ephemerida larvae	1.5
		Notonecta sp.	1.5
		Chironomus plumosus	1.5
Chordata	Pisces	Carassius carassius	3
	Amphibia	Triton taeniatus	1.5
		Larvae of Rana temporaria	1.5

Twice or thrice the lethal dose of the drug was given internally to the animal. Immediately after respiratory arrest or — in the experiments with santonin — after the appearance of the first signs of poisoning, blood was taken from the heart for determination of the concentration of the drug. The blood was stabilized with citrate. In the experiments with volatile substances — carbon tetrachloride and tetrachloroethylene — the animals were poisoned by the inhalation route. In these experiments the blood sample was taken soon after the cessation of breathing.

The anthelminthic substances in the blood were estimated quantitatively by means of a type SF-4 quartz spectrophotometer. The blood sample was shaken for 10 minutes with twice its volume of solvent. The solvent was then separated by centrifugation and examined photometrically in rectangular dishes, 1 cm thick, using selected key waves.

The substances were identified qualitatively by the shape of the absorption spectrograms (Fig. 3); their concentration was calculated by means of the formula:

$$C = \frac{DV_p f \cdot 10^5}{kdV_k} \text{ mg\%,}$$

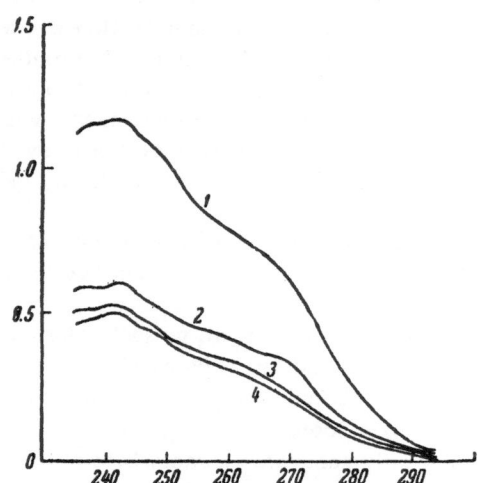

Fig. 3. Absorption spectrogram of a solution of santonin in dichloroethane (1) and of dichloroethane extracts of the blood of rabbits poisoned with santonin (2-4). Along the axis of abscissas — wavelength (mμ); along the axis of ordinates — optical density.

where C is the concentration in mg%; D is the optical density; V_p is the volume of solvent in ml; V_k is the volume of blood in ml; f is the correction factor for incomplete extraction; k is the coefficient of absorption at the key wavelength, in $cm^2 g^{-1}$ (Table 5); d is the thickness of the dish in cm; 10^5 is the coefficient of conversion from g/ml to mg%.

Contamination of the test samples in a pilot experiment was insignificant and was disregarded. In the experiments with santonin, the following toxic manifestions were observed after administration of the drug: salivation, rigidity of movements, tremor, spasms, loud and anxious mewing, and attacks of fits or vomiting. During the fits, which were tonicoclonic in character, the animal lay on its belly with its paws wide apart. The blood sample was taken shortly after the appearance of one of the signs of poisoning (the first to develop).

TABLE 5. Key Waves, Coefficients of Absorption of Ultraviolet Light, and Extraction of Substances from the Blood in Percent

Substance	Solvent	Key wave, mμ (λ)	Coefficient of absorption (k)	% extraction	Correction factor for incomplete extraction (f)
Hexylresorcinol	Dichloroethane	280	13595	80	1.25
Thymol	Dichloroethane	275	15000	105	0.95
Tetrachloroethylene	Hexane	235	17400	80	1.25
Carbon tetrachloride	Hexane	220	732	92	1.09
Santonin	Dichloroethane	260	33900	99	1.01

The toxic action of oxygen could be observed only when it acted under pressure. As Baer (1878, cited by Lazarev, 1941) first showed, oxygen causes strychnine-like convulsions in animals. A cat was placed in a high-pressure chamber with a volume of 60 liters. A chemical absorbent was present in the chamber to remove CO_2. After closure of the hatch, pure oxygen was passed into the chamber for 2-5 minutes, and the pressure was then raised by giving oxygen from a balloon. When two hours had elapsed, a sample of gas was taken from the chamber for determination of the partial pressure of oxygen and carbon dioxide. The pressure was then lowered to atmospheric and the cat taken from the chamber. If the cat died before the two hours had elapsed, the sampling and decompression were carried out immediately after death. We give below an extract from the records of one of the experiments with oxygen.

9:10 AM	Cat weighing 2.52 kg placed in high-pressure chamber. Chamber closed. Ventilation with pure oxygen carried out.
9:12 AM	Compression begun.
9:15 AM	Pressure raised to 6.0 absolute atmospheres. Animal's condition normal.
9:32 AM	Cat looks anxiously for the way out.
9:36 AM	Convulsions of a clonicotonic character.
9:37 AM	Lies down and mews.
9:39 AM	Second attack of convulsions lasting 0.5 minute.
9:42 AM to 9:47 AM	Nine severe convulsions, separated by short intervals.
9:47 AM to 10:20 AM	Convulsions repeated several times a minute, gradually becoming weaker.
10:28 AM	Coma. Isolated convulsive spasms.
10:33 AM	Breathing irregular.
10:50 AM	Breathing ceased. Death. Sample of gas taken from the chamber. Results of analysis in Orsat's apparatus: oxygen 97%, carbon dioxide 0.4%. Partial pressure of oxygen 5.82 atm. Death took place after 1 hr 35 min.

In 2 of the 7 experiments, the cat died. Death did not occur when the pressure was less than 5.62 atm. This result agrees with the findings of Behnke (cited by Lazarev, 1941): convulsions developed as a rule in the animals if the partial pressure of oxygen exceeded 5 atm. In response to the action of the other substances, death took place during profound narcosis.

The lethal or toxic concentrations of hexylresorcinol, carbon tetrachloride, thymol, tetrachloroethylene, santonin, and oxygen established in the experiments on cats, and of some of these substances in experiments on rabbits, are given in Table 7.

3. The Toxic Concentrations of Anthelminthic Substances for Toxocara

Helminths of the genus Toxocara were obtained from the intestines of cats killed by electrocution. The helminths were placed in Ringer's solution warmed to 38°, and were used in the experiments on the same day.

The toxicity of oxygen was determined by passing a current of gas through the Ringer's solution in which the helminths were kept. When oxygen was passed at a pressure equal to atmospheric, the helminths became immobile and died two hours after the beginning of the experiment.

TABLE 6. The Toxic Action of Some Anthelminthic Substances on Toxocara and Ascaris

Substance	Toxic action on Toxocara (figures from Paribok, 1955,1957)			Toxic action on Ascaris		
	Toxic concentration (in mg%)		Duration of exposure	Toxic concentration (in mg%)	Duration of exposure	Author
	in the medium	in the body of the helminth				
Hexylresorcinol	—	41	A few minutes	1-10	24 hr	Krotov (1953)
				50	1-2 hr	Varlakov (1939)
				100	1-2 min	Lamson et al. (1935a)
Thymol	—	90	The same	20	2 hr	Varlakov (1939)
				12	2 hr	Oelkers (1943)
				30	1.5 hr	Brüning (cited by Oelkers, 1943)
Tetrachloroethylene	—	138	" "	70	2 hr	Oelkers (1943)
Carbon tetrachloride	—	118-166	" "	80	less than 2 hr	
Santonin	0.5	—	" "	more than 0.00001	?	Kobayachi et al. (1952)
Oxygen (in abs. atm.)	1	—	2 hr	1	2 hr	Kravets (1953)

Immobility of the helminths was also the criterion of toxicity of the action of hexylresorcinol, thymol, tetrachloroethylene, and carbon tetrachloride. Helminths were placed in solutions of the anthelminthic drugs and extracted at the moment when they ceased to move, when they were rinsed three times with distilled water, dried with filter paper, weighed on torsion scales, and transferred to the vessels containing the solvents. The same solvents were used as in the experiments on the cats and rabbits. Three days later the optical density of the hexane or dichloroethane extracts was determined by ultraviolet photometry.

Control investigations showed that the solvents extract rather more extraneous matter from the bodies of the helminths than from the animals' blood. A suitable correction was accordingly introduced into the calculations.

Santonin does not cause death and does not immobilize nematodes (Baldwin, 1948; Krotov, 1958). In the experiments with santonin we therefore registered the appearance of the first signs of poisoning in the helminths. (It will be remembered that in the experiments on cats,also,the initial signs of poisoning were registered.) These took the form of spasms of the helminths, which curled into a tight spiral resembling a spring. In a solution of santonin with a concentration of 0.5 mg% these signs of poisoning appeared after 3-5 minutes. In view of the fact that the content of santonin in the bodies of the helminths was extremely small, photometry of the extracts was impracticable, and the estimated concentration of santonin in the solution is shown subsequently.

The values of the toxicity of the anthelminthics obtained in these experiments were compared with the findings of other workers (Table 6). Attention must be drawn to the following circumsance: In the papers cited, the concentration of anthelminthics is given not in the body of the helminths,but in the surrounding fluid. Theoretically this method is above reproach, for the measure of toxicity must be regarded as the concentration of the substance in the medium and not in the cells. The difficulty which arises when the experiments are performed in this way is that it is not easy to determine beforehand the necessary duration of observation. From the example of hexylresorcinol (Table 6) it may be seen that the concentrations of poison causing the same effect for 24 hours, 1-2 hours, or 1-2 minutes differ widely. It is therefore still uncertain what concentration to use as lethal.

If the concentration of the anthelminthic is determined in the body of the helminth and not in the medium, this difficulty does not arise, for the experiment finishes at the moment of appearance of the effect in which the experimenter is interested (the same applied in the experiments on cats and rabbits). We may thus compare the toxic concentrations of the group of substances for Toxocara established in our experiments with the toxic concentrations for Ascaris.

The toxic concentration of hexylresorcinol for Toxocara lies within the limits which characterize its toxicity for Ascaris. The somewhat higher values of the concentrations of thymol, tetrachloroethylene, and carbon tetrachloride may be explained by differences in the duration of exposure (the experiments on Toxocara lasted only a few minutes, while those on Ascaris lasted 2 hours). At a pressure of 1 atm, oxygen has a toxic action on both Ascaris

TABLE 7. The Toxicity of Anthelminthics for Cats, Rabbits, and Toxocara (Paribok. 1956)

| Substance | Action on higher animals | | A | | Action on Toxocara | A | B | | Ratio B/A |
	Criterion of toxic action	Species of animal	Concentration of substance in blood (mg%)	Partial pressure of substance in medium (atm)	Criterion of toxic action	Concentration of substance in body of helminths (mg%)	Concentration of substance in medium (mg%)	Partial pressure of substance in medium (atm)	
Hexylresorcinol	Death	Cats	4.4	–	Immobilization	41	–	–	9.3
Thymol	"	"	10.0	–	The same	90	–	–	9.0
Carbon tetrachloride	"	"	37.0	–	The same	144 (118–166)	–	–	3.9
Tetrachloroethylene	"	"	10.5	–	The same	138	–	–	13
Carbon tetrachloride	"	Rabbits	58.0	–	–	–	–	–	–
Tetrachloroethylene	"	"	18.5	–	–	–	–	–	–
Santonin	Initial signs of poisoning	Cats	2.7	–	Initial signs of poisoning	–	less than 0.5	–	less than 0.18
Oxygen	Death within 2 hr	"	–	5.7	Death	–	–	1	0.18

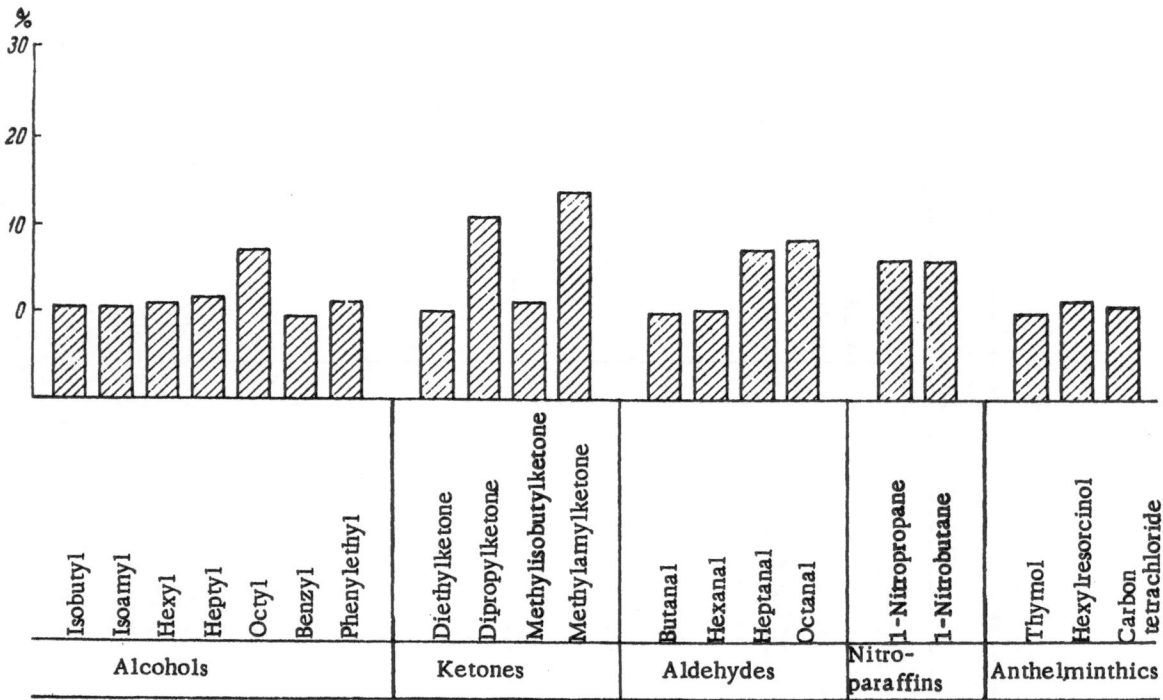

Fig. 4. Thermodynamic toxic concentrations of nonelectrolytes for <u>Cosmocerca ornata</u>. The concentrations are expressed as percentages of the solubility of the substances in water.

and Toxocara, and causes death of these helminths within 2 hours. In the experiments on Toxocara, santonin was tested in concentrations of not less than 0.5 mg%. According to Kobayachi et al. (1952), the character of movement of Ascaris is disturbed by even smaller concentrations of santonin. The results of these experiments thus agree in the main with those reported in the literature.

In Table 7 we summarize the results of experiments to determine the toxicity of anthelminthics for cats, rabbits, and helminths of the genus Toxocara. The last column shows the ratio between the toxic concentrations for the nematodes and the toxic concentrations for the host. <u>In the case of the first four anthelminthics — hexylresorcinol, thymol, carbon tetrachloride, and tetrachloroethylene — this ratio is greater than unity.</u> Consequently, these anthelminthics are less toxic to the helminths than to the host.

In contrast to these, santonin and oxygen have a weaker action on the host than on the helminths: the ratio between the toxic concentrations here is less than unity. Of the total number of anthelminthics tested, thus only santonin and oxygen are characterized by a ratio between toxicity to parasite and toxicity to host (the etiotropic property is stronger than the organotropic) such as obtains in a typical chemotherapeutic substance: in antibiotics and sulfonamides.

The first four substances exhibit a peculiar "chemotherapeutic paradox", for their <u>organotropic</u> action is stronger than their <u>etiotropic</u> action.

4. Comparison Between the Toxicity Toward the Nematode Cosmocerca ornata of Anthelminthic Drugs with a Nonelectrolytic Action and Other Narcotics

One method of elucidating the mechanism of the toxic action of any substance is to compare the character and strength of its action with the character and strength of the action of more fully investigated substances on the same object. The "strength of action" of the substance may be expressed most accurately as the concentration in the presence of which the biological effect in which the experimenter is interested takes place. In the case of nonelectrolytes, the acting concentrations of the substances may change a thousandfold (compare Fig. 1).

When comparing the concentrations of nonelectrolytes causing the desired effect with the iso-effective concentrations of substances whose mechanism of action is being investigated, it would therefore be necessary in both cases to take into account the physicochemical properties of these substances and to introduce the appropriate corrections. The corrections may be introduced automatically, if the concentration of the substances is expressed not

TABLE 8. Toxic Concentrations of Various Compounds for the Meal Worm (Albert, 1953)

Substance	Toxic concentration at 15° (μmoles/liter)	Thermodynamic concentration
Monomethylaniline	3.7	0.3
Dimethylaniline	6.6	0.4
Pyridine	76	0.1
Bromoform	94	0.5
Bromobenzene	96	0.7
Tetrachloroethane	141	0.6
Chlorobenzene	200	0.5
p-Xylene	230	0.6
Toluene	420	0.4
Nitromethane	710	0.6
Benzene	775	0.2
Heptane	800	0.5
Chloroform	1040	0.2
Carbon tetrachloride	1600	0.4
Trichloroethylene	1200	0.4
Hexane	3000	0.6
Dichloroethane	3100	0.2
Pentane	16000	0.9

in absolute units, but, employing Ferguson's (1939) suggestion, as a ratio between the acting concentration and the solubility of the substance in water (see also Albert, 1953, p. 37). This value is called the thermodynamic concentration. If the substance does not act in solution but as a vapor. it is expressed as the quotient obtained by dividing the vapor pressure at which the toxic effect takes place by the vapor pressure at that particular temperature.

Ferguson showed that the numerical values of this index — the thermodynamic concentration or, alternatively, the relative saturation of the toxic concentration–for substances acting nonspecifically (as narcotics) on the selected object are very close, and as a rule the largest is not more than ten times greater than the smallest (Table 8).

This conclusion may also be drawn from what we already know of the pattern of action of the nonelectrolytes and its relationship to their physicochemical properties (see Chapter 1). If the solubility in water and the acting concentrations (for example, narcotic) of a series of nonelectrolytes undergo parallel changes, the ratio between these values will not vary very considerably from one compound to another.

From the foregoing facts we may draw the following conclusion. By determining the toxicity of a series of compounds with nonelectrolytic action, and expressing it in the form of thermodynamic concentrations, we may obtain a criterion (a "standard") for assessing the action of any other substance on the same object. If the ratio between the toxic concentration and the solubility of the test substance (the thermodynamic concentration) is close to that for substances of known nonelectrolytic action, it may be assumed that the mechanism of action is the same in both cases. In the opposite case, i.e., if this ratio is appreciably smaller than the established "standard," it must be concluded that the mechanism of action of the substance is specific, and different from nonelectrolytic.

In view of these considerations, the following experiments were carried out. We investigated the toxicity toward the nematode Cosmocerca ornata of a series of nonelectrolytes (alcohols, aldehydes, etc.), and also of certain anthelminthic drugs. The nematodes were obtained from the intestine of a frog, and placed in batches of ten in glass vessels. The experiments with volatile substances, the concentration of which might fall rapidly during work in open glass vessels, were conducted in special miniature vessels with ground stoppers.

The results were treated by the method of summation of frequencies. The concentration at which 50 percent of the helminths were rendered immobile was determined by interpolation and expressed as a percentage of the solubility of the substance in water.

Experiments were conducted with twenty different compounds, including alcohols, ketones, aldehydes, nitroparaffins, and three anthelminthic drugs: thymol, carbon tetrachloride, and hexylresorcinol. It was found that the thermodynamic toxic concentrations of the anthelminthics lie within the limits of variation of concentration of the remaining nonelectrolytes (Fig. 4).

The suggestion that all the substances tested could produce some special (not narcotic) effect, connected by a simple relationship with the solubility of the substances, appears unlikely. The mechanism of action in these cases is undoubtedly nonelectrolytic. Consequently, the action of the anthelminthics tested in these experiments must also be regarded as a nonelectrolytic effect.

Chapter 3

THE PRINCIPLE AND METHOD OF TRIAL OF ANTHELMINTHIC AND ANTIPROTOZOAL COMPOUNDS WITH NONELECTROLYTIC ACTION

The evidence of the nonelectrolytic mechanism of action of anthelminthic compounds (carbon tetrachloride and others) given in the preceding chapter would be of no real importance if the number of anthelminthic drugs acting in this manner were limited to the few existing preparations. Can we not expect to find new anthelminthics with a nonelectrolytic action, which will be more effective than the existing preparations? Is it not possible to obtain a combination of suitable properties in a particular case: a strong nonelectrolytic action and, consequently, high toxicity toward helminths, combined with low solubility and slow absorption from the alimentary tract, and the ability to be excreted rapidly through the lungs or kidneys — properties characteristic of carbon tetrachloride, hexylresorcinol, and related substances — or are these properties unique and irreproducible?

In order to ascertain the gravity of the risk, we must examine the manner in which, on the one hand, the toxicity of nonelectrolytes toward helminths, and on the other, their ability to undergo absorption in the intestine and, consequently, their toxicity toward animals when administered via the gastrointestinal tract, are dependent on the physicochemical properties of these compounds. This would enable it to be established to what extent the suitable combination of these properties in the existing anthelminthics with nonelectrolytic action is typical.

The anser to the first of these questions was given earlier (Chapter 1): in a series of nonelectrolytes arranged in order of decreasing solubility in water, the toxicity toward helminths, like the action on other biological objects found in an aqueous medium, increases. The second question calls for a special examination.

1. The Toxicity of Nonelectrolytes When Administered Internally

Let us consider how the toxicity of nonelectrolytes changes within the limits of a given homologous series. Lamson, Brown, and Ward (1935a) investigated the ascaricidal action and toxicity of polyhydroxybenzene compounds toward rats. Whereas the maximum of ascaricidal action was observed with hexylresorcinol, the most toxic compound toward rats was the first member of the series, namely resorcinol, and the higher homologs had a much weaker action. Lamson and co-workers (1935b) obtained similar results in experiments with orthoalkylphenols. In this series of compounds, o-butylphenol showed the strongest ascaricidal action (in a concentration of 1:1000); the toxicity of the alkyl-substituted phenols toward rats decreased from the first member of the series to the subsequent members (Table 9).

The toxicity of the alkyl-m-cresols when introduced into the gastrointestinal tract of animals also decreases with lengthening of their hydrocarbon radical (Lamson and Brown, 1935c). At first sight these facts openly disagree with the well-known principle, first discovered by Richardson (1869, cited by Lazarev, 1940) and subsequently confirmed on many occasions: the increased biological activity of nonelectrolytes in a homologous series when passing from the lower homologs to the higher.

The reason for this disagreement lies in the special conditions of action of poisons introduced into the gastrointestinal tract, which differ from those applying in experiments on organisms completely immersed in an aqueous solution of the poison. When they enter the gastrointestinal tract, nonelectrolytes are partially dissolved in the intestinal contents and are then absorbed. The rate of absorption of nonelectrolytes from solutions of equal concentration (equimolar) in a series of compounds increases with the lengthening of the hydrocarbon radical.[*] Lengthening of

---

[*]In relation to helminths, this principle was established by Trim for the alkylresorcinols. It also applies when nonelectrolytes are introduced into other biological objects (see Lazarev, 1944b, p. 120).

TABLE 9. Toxicity of o-Alkylphenols toward Rats (Injected into the Stomach through a Tube). Data of Lamson et al. (1935b)

Compound	Dose causing death of 50% of animals (in mg/kg)
Phenol	0.3
o-n-Butylphenol	0.65
o-n-Amylphenol	0.70
o-n-Hexylphenol	1.30
o-n-Heptylphenol	2.75
o-n-Octylphenol	2.80

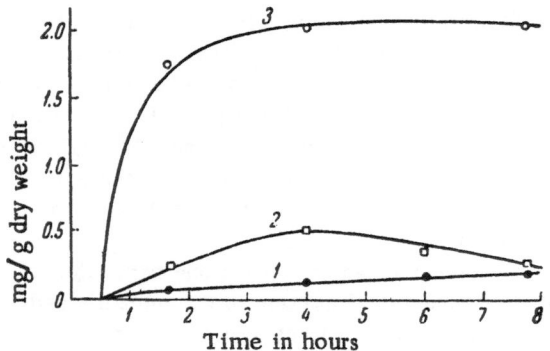

Fig. 5. Phenothiazine content in the blood (1) and intestinal mucosa (2) of a chick and in the bodies of nematodes (Ascaridia galli) (3) inhabiting its intestine (Lasarus and Rogers, 1951).

the hydrocarbon radical is accompanied, however, by another phenomenon: the solubility of the compounds in water decreases. Since the determination of toxic substances requires their internal administration, not as equimolecular aqueous solutions, but in the form of suspensions, emulsions, or in the undiluted state, the decrease in solubility in homologous series essentially modifies the conditions of absorption of the compounds from the intestine. Under these circumstances the concentrations of the substances in true aqueous solution in the intestine are not equal.

The higher homologs which, under identical conditions (in equal concentrations of their aqueous solutions), would be absorbed more rapidly, are less soluble and are therefore present in smaller concentrations than the lower members of the series — readily soluble, but more slowly absorbed substances. Hence, it follows that the potentially more toxic substances are in fact (when administered internally) less toxic because of their insufficient solubility. This leads to an apparent infringement of Richardson's rule.

If all these arguments are valid, the question arises why, in a homologous series of substances, during the passage from the lower homologs to the higher, the action of the compounds on mammals only, and not on helminths, is weakened? The parasites are apparently in the same conditions as the intestinal wall, for they are exposed to the action of the poison in the same concentration.

Although the conditions of absorption are, in fact, the same as a first approximation, considerable differences exist in the conditions of elimination of the poison. The helminths are completely immersed in the poison solution and their entire body surface is in contact with it. However slowly the poison entered, provided that its concentration in the medium was adequate, saturation of the helminths must take place, for the poison could be "excreted nowhere."

The fate of the poison in the body of the host is different. After absorption from the intestine it enters the portal vein and the lymphatics. The poison may be partly retained by the liver and returned to the intestine or neutralized. We may mention in passing that the circulation of the poison through the system, portal vein–biliary tract, is important in the case of its action on liver helminths (see Chapter 7).

The minute volume of the blood flow in the intestinal vessels is about 25% of that in the general circulation (Spector, 1956). The poison entering the postcaval vein has thus been diluted more than fourfold.

Lasarus and Rogers (1951) introduced phenothiazine into the stomach of chicks and then determined its content in the bodies of helminths (Ascaridia galli, inhabiting the intestine of chicks), and in the tissue of the intestinal mucous membrane and the blood of the chicks. The concentration of the poison in the blood was several times less than in the bodies of the helminths (Fig. 5).

When they pass through the pulmonary vessels, certain poisons with a low coefficient of solubility of their vapor in water and blood, i.e., which pass readily from blood to air, are rapidly excreted through the lungs. Their concentration in the arterial blood thus falls much lower. For example, when a saturated solution of tetrachloroethylene is passed through an area of bowel, the concentration of the compound in the arterial blood is less than one-tenth of that in the intestine, and in some experiments no tetrachloroethylene can be detected in the arterial blood (Fig. 10). It is thus perfectly practicable to obtain a ratio between the rates of absorption and excretion of the poison at which its concentration in the intestine will be high, thereby producing a toxic action on the helminths, and its concentration in the blood low, and thereby harmless to the host.

We may compare the toxicity of certain nonelectrolyes when introduced into the gastrointestinal tract with their solubility in water (Fig. 6). The solubility of 25 compounds, the values of which were used in plotting the graph, shows a difference of 1400 times between the extreme variants (the distance between the extreme left and right

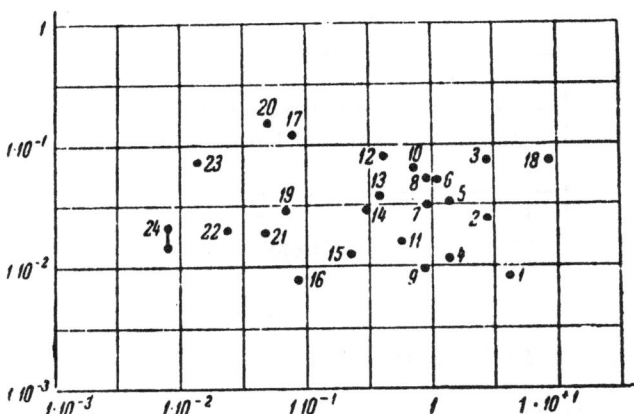

Fig. 6. Solubility of nonelectrolytes in water and their toxicity after internal administration to albino rats. Along the axis of abscissas — solubility in water (moles per liter); along the axis of ordinates — LD_{50} for rats (moles per kg). Compounds: 1) chloral hydrate; 2) propionaldehyde; 3) secondary butyl alcohol; 4) amylene hydrate; 5) isobutyl alcohol; 6) iso-oleic aldehyde; 7) ethyl acetoacetate; 8) butyl alcohol; 9) phenol; 10) ethyl acetate; 11) diethyl ketone; 12) n-oleic aldehyde; 13) orthocresol; 14) isopropyl acetate; 15) acetaldehyde; 16) ethylene chloride; 17) butyl acetate; 18) dioxan; 19) chloroform; 20) dichloroethane; 21) metacresol; 22) 1,2-dichloropropane; 23) benzene; 24) n-heptyl alcohol.

points); the difference between the lethal doses* is only 18 times (the distance from the top to the bottom points). In this case, there is no clear pattern of change of toxicity of a homologous series of compounds when administered internally (see Table 9), for the results presented here relate to compounds belonging to different homologous series. It is obvious, however, that compounds of low toxicity may be encountered among nonelectrolytes which are both readily and poorly soluble in water.

We pointed out above that if the toxicity of substances toward objects totally immersed in aqueous solutions of nonelectrolytes is investigated, a different pattern is observed. As the solubility of the nonelectrolytes in water decreases, their toxicity increases regularly. If we compare this phenomenon with the fact that, in a series of nonelectrolytes arranged in order of decreasing solubility in water, little change is found in the toxicity of the compounds when administered internally, we may conclude that substances possessing suitable properties for anthelminthic action should be sought among nonelectrolytes with poor solubility in water. The existing anthelminthic drugs with nonelectrolytic action are not the only compounds of this type, and there is every reason to suppose that others may be discovered with equally or, perhaps, more suitable combinations of properties.

2. The Method of Trial of Anthelminthic Drugs with Nonelectrolytic Action

The basis for clinical trial of new anthelminthic drugs, as with other chemotherapeutic preparations, is the positive results of treatment in experiments with infested animals. Such model infestation experiments are not, however, the first step in the search for suitable drugs. The investigation, on such models, of all substances with suspected chemotherapeutic activity that could be produced on theoretical grounds would involve an enormous expenditure of effort and time, and it would delay the prospects of success. Moreover, many of the substances originally chosen would subsequently have to be discarded because of their low efficacy or high toxicity. It is therefore desirable and, as a rule, necessary to use pilot methods of selection of compounds for further experimental-therapeutic trial, employing simple methods such as are used in trials of antibiotics or other antibacterial agents. These experiments exclude at once those compounds with little or no activity.

Experiments in vitro may lead to the omission from further investigation of compounds which aquire chemotherapeutic activity as a result of transformation within the body of the host. In the case of anthelminthic substances with nonelectrolytic action, however (the effect of which, like other nonelectrolytic effects such as narcosis, is not related to their ability to take part in chemical reactions, i.e., does not depend on conversion within the body or, in particular, in the intestine), there is no danger of any such omission.

By experiments in vitro the most active compounds, i.e., those acting on the test object in the lowest concentrations, will be selected for further investigation. Before starting an experimental therapeutic investigation it is also desirable to determine the toxicity of a preparation exhibiting activity in experiments in vitro by introducing it into the gastrointestinal tract of animals. Some doubt may be expressed on this point, for the following reason. Let us assume that a certain test substance in experiments in vitro causes death of helminths in a concentration of 0.01 g/liter, and that its lethal dose for the animal when administered internally is 0.5 g/kg. Is this good or bad? Can it be expected that this substance will have an anthelminthic action in experiments on animals? It is impossible to answer this question on the basis of these hypothetical considerations alone, without other data.

The situation is changed radically if the experimenter, having obtained such information, compares it with the action on helminths and the toxicity toward higher animals of anthelminthics already known and in use, which

_____

* Data on the toxicity of compounds taken from Spector's handbook (Spector, 1956); data on the solubility in water of compounds 2, 3, 6, 7, 11, and 12 from the Handbook of Physical and Chemical Values, Technical Encyclopedia (1931), Vol. 4; solubility of the remaining compounds according to data from Lazarev's book (Lazarev, 1944b, 1954).

TABLE 10.

Hypothetical preparations	Lethal dose when administered internally, g/kg (LD)	Lethal concentration for helminths, g/liter (LC_{50})	$\dfrac{LD}{LC_{50}}$	Conclusion regarding the value of further tests
Standard	0.3	0.03	10	–
No. 1	0.5	0.01	50	Useful
No. 2	0.05	0.002	25	Useful
No. 3	0.3	0.6	0.5	Useless

TABLE 11. Minimal Lethal Doses of Nonelectrolytes for Albino Mice, and Concentrations Immobilizing 50% of Nematodes

Substance	LC_{50} (in millimoles per liter)	MLD (in millimoles per kg)	$K = \dfrac{MLD}{LC_{50}}$
Methyl alcohol	1960	353	0.18
Ethyl alcohol	920	217	0.24
Urethane	520	84.2	0.16
Ethyl acetate	111	45.4	0.41
Isobutyl alcohol	70	67.2	0.95
Guaiacol	22	9	0.41
Chloroform	3.4	8.6	2.5
Thymol	0.55	3.4	6.2
Carbon tetrachloride	0.51	20.0	39
Hexylresorcinol	0.27	2.0	7.5

he adopts as a "standard." If the corresponding figures obtained for the new substance are of the same order as those for existing anthelminthics, the new compound should be tested on animals. For example, if it were known beforehand that the lethal dose of the "standard preparation" is 0.3 g/kg and its toxic concentration for helminths 0.03 g per liter, it is obvious that this particular hypothetical preparation (with corresponding figures of 5 g/kg and 0.01 g per liter) should be tested further.

What is the position regarding another hypothetical preparation with higher toxicity than the standard (for example, 0.05 g/kg) and also with higher activity (active concentration on helminths 0.002 g/liter)? It would obviously be useful here to calculate the ratio between the toxic dose for the animal and the effective concentration (active on the parasite), for the chemotherapeutic efficacy of the preparation is more, probably, the lower its toxicity toward the host (high lethal dose when administered internally) and the stronger its action on the parasite (low lethal concentration toward helminths).

$$\frac{\text{lethal dose on internal administration}}{\text{lethal concentration toward helminths}} = \frac{LD}{LC_{50}}$$

We give below the results of this calculation in the case of a standard and three hypothetical new substances, two of which have been mentioned above (Table 10).

It will be clear from Table 10 that trials of the first and second hypothetical substances, for which the ratio LD/LC_{50} is greater than for the standard preparation, are desirable, whereas the third preparation is inferior to the standard and it would be useless to test it further.

In view of the foregoing considerations, we have developed the following method of selection of suggested anthelminthic substances for subsequent experimental therapeutic investigation in animals (Paribok, 1952). The action of the substances on helminths was investigated on the nematode Cosmocerca ornata, obtained from the intestine of the frog. The method described in the previous chapter was adopted: the concentrations of the substances in each particular case were expressed not as a fraction of the concentration of the saturated solution, but in milligrams or millimoles per liter. Substances with no action on the nematode were excluded from further investigation. The toxicity of the remaining substances (i.e., those which immobilized the nematode in a certain concentration) was determined by experiments on mice. The substances were introduced into the stomach of the mouse through a tube and their minimal lethal doses were ascertained.

TABLE 12. Narcotic Concentrations of Ether and Chloroform for Protozoa and Helminths (according to Makarov, 1938)

Object	Narcotic concentrations (in moles/liter)	
	ether	chloroform
Protozoa		
Opalina ranarum	0.27	0.012
Vorticella	0.34	0.006
Colpidium colpoda	0.20	0.006
Balantidium	0.20	0.012
Helminths		
Rhabditis sp.	0.20	0.012
Polystomum sp.	0.20	—
Dolychosaccus rastellus	0.20	0.012
Haplometra cilindrocoelum	0.20	0.012

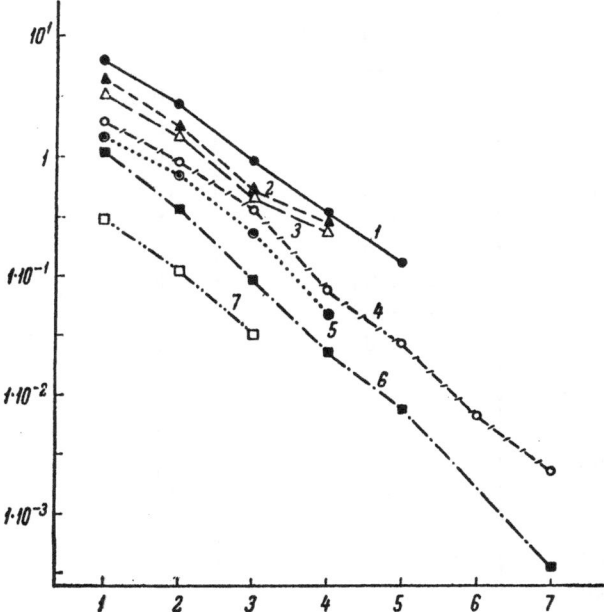

Fig. 7. Various forms of nonelectrolytic action in a series of monoatomic alcohols. Along the axis of abscissas — number of carbon atoms in the alcohol molecule; along the axis of ordinates — concentrations causing corresponding effects (moles/liter): 1) hemolysis; decreased staining power of muscle; 3) depression of electrical excitability of muscle; 4) immobilization of Cosmocerca ornata; 5) immobilization of Paramecium caudatum; 6) narcosis of fishes; 7) narcosis of tadpoles.

In order to discover the values of the lethal doses and the corresponding lethal concentrations of the standard preparations, preliminary experiments were conducted with thymol, carbon tetrachloride, and hexylresorcinol. For purposes of comparison in this series of experiments we determined the toxicity toward mice and helminths of a series of nonelectrolytes having no anthelminthic action. In Table 11, in which we give the results of these experiments, we also give the calculated values of the coefficients MLD/LC_{50}.

The value of the coefficient is very characteristic. Whereas for the alcohols and other compounds with no anthelminthic action the coefficient is less than unity, for the anthelminthics of nonelectrolytic action, including chloroform, it is greater than unity. In Table 11 the substances are arranged in order of decreasing solubility in water. It will be evident that the toxic concentrations for nematodes decrease to a far greater degree than the minimal lethal doses as the solubility decreases, which is responsible for a change in the coefficient MLD/LC_{50} from fractional values (substances in the upper half of the table) to whole numbers (lower half).

It may thus be concluded that by determining this coefficient for other substances not previously studied for their anthelminthic activity, the most promising of them may be selected for further experimental therapeutic investigation.

According to Makarov (1938), narcosis of helminths is cellular and paranecrotic in nature. The strength of action of narcotics on different organisms characterized by general narcosis of cellular type differs only very little (Table 12).

In view of these facts, should other organisms besides nematodes be used in trials of new anthelminthics with nonelectrolytic action?

Zakabunin (1949) introduced into the gastrointestinal tract of albino mice many nonelectrolytes, the toxic concentrations of which toward infusoria (Paramecium caudatum) had previously been determined (Paribok, 1945), and ascertained their toxicity toward these animals. The substances tested included narcotics with no anthelminthic action and also typical anthelminthic nonelectrolytes. The same pattern was observed when infusoria were used as in the experiments with nematodes. The value of the coefficient MLD/LC_{50} for the anthelminthics was higher than for the other substances (Table 13), and it also exceeded unity.

Other biological objects could also have been used in these pilot experiments. The coincidence between their sensitivity to narcotics and the sensitivity of parasitic helminths to these narcotics, so strange at first sight, is not of decisive importance. The fact is that the concentrations of nonelectrolytes at which particular biological effects (narcosis of vertebrate animals, immobilization of parasitic helminths or infusoria, hemolysis) arise bear approximately

TABLE 13. Toxic Concentrations for Paramecium (LC_{50}), Minimal Lethal Doses for Albino Mice when Administered Enterally (MLD), and Coefficients MLD/LC_{50} (Zakabunin, 1949)

Substance	LC_{50} (in millimoles per liter)	MLD (in millimoles per kg)	$K = \dfrac{MLD}{LC_{50}}$
Methyl alcohol	1400	< 700	< 0.5
Ethyl alcohol	700	< 350	< 0.5
Urethane	285	< 142	< 0.5
Dioxan	250	< 125	< 0.5
Isopropyl alcohol	245	< 122	< 0.5
Ethyl alcohol	214	< 107	< 0.5
Trimethylcarbinol	126	< 63	< 0.5
Ethyl acetoacetate	126	< 63	< 0.5
Ethyl acetate	118	< 59	< 0.5
Triacetine	74	< 37	< 0.5
Ethyl bromide	60	< 30	< 0.5
Isobutyl alcohol	47	< 47	< 1.0
Pyramidon	34	< 17	< 0.5
Caffeine	33	< 16.5	< 0.5
Acetanilide	29	< 14.5	< 0.5
Chloral hydrate	27.1	< 13.5	< 0.5
Guaiacol	18	< 9	< 0.5
Dial	17.6	< 8.8	< 0.5
Methylene chloride	14.8	< 7.2	< 0.5
Coumarin	14.4	< 7.2	< 0.5
Chloroform	8.6	8.6	1
Bromural	8.1	< 4.05	< 0.5
Chloretone	7.75	< 3.87	< 0.5
Ethylene bromide	6.59	< 6.59	< 1
Paraldehyde	6.3	< 6.3	< 1
Avertin	5.75	< 5.75	< 1
Benzene	4.6	32.2	7
Ethyl iodide	4.5	< 2.25	< 0.5
Carbon tetrachloride	0.85	20	22
Menthol	0.83	< 0.41	< 0.5
Beta-naphthol	0.44	4.1	9
Thymol	0.34	3.4	10
Hexylresorcinol	0.052	2	38

the same relationship in different substances (Fig. 7).[*] In other words, if, for example, the narcotic concentration of one substance is twice that of another, the hemolytic concentrations will bear the same relationship. If, therefore, we replace one object by another, although we obtain a different value for the coefficient LD/LC_{50}, the fundamental principle still holds good, i.e., the value of the coefficient is high in the case of substances with anthelminthic activity.

This conclusion might have been anticipated in view of the nonspecific, nonelectrolytic mechanism of the anthelminthic action of carbon tetrachloride and similar anthelminthic compounds. If, in fact, the anthelminthic effect of these substances were due to a suitable correlation between strong nonelectrolytic action and low toxicity when administered internally (weak absorption and rapid excretion), then in the trial of new substances of this type the aim

---

[*] Source of data: Hemolytic concentrations — Fühner; narcotic concentrations for tadpoles — Overton; narcotic concentrations for fishes — Lendle (cited by Lazarev, 1940); concentrations causing decreased staining power and depression of electrical excitability of muscle — Nasonov and Aleksandrov (1940); concentrations immobilizing Paramecium and the nematode Cosmocerca ornata — Paribok (1945, 1952).

must be to discover in some way these characteristics of the substance. Since the nonelectrolytic action is exhibited in experiments with various biological objects, not only helminths but also other organisms or cells may be used for their detection.

The views expressed in this chapter do not agree, at first sight, with the generally accepted ideas of the methods of trial of anthelminthics, but they appear to be directly contradictory. Attempts to use nonparasitic worms and other animals to study the action of anthelminthics have often been made. Straub (1902, cited by Shul'ts and Shikhobalova, 1934) and, later, Varlakov (1939) investigated the mechanism of action of anthelminthic drugs in experiments on earthworms. Geckelberg (1888), Trendelenburg (1916), and Joachimoglu and Bose (1924, cited by Shul'ts and Shikhobalova, 1934) used leeches for this purpose. For the biological assay of male fern preparations in accordance with the standard of the International Hygiene Committee, the use of small fishes has been suggested. Careful confirmatory investigations (see literature cited by Shul'ts and Shikhobalova, 1934) led, however, to the abandonment of these and most similar test objects. The main reason for this abandonment was the discrepancy between the concentrations causing immobilization of helminths and the concentrations of the same substances having a toxic action on other objects. In the experiments of Lamson and Ward (1936), agreement between the toxic concentrations for <u>Ascaris suis</u> and the earthworm was found in only 6% of investigations.

In the case of a substance with a specific mechanism of its anthelminthic action, the use of biological objects other than parasitic worms for selection is in fact undesirable and incorrect. Specific anthelminthic substances of the type of santonin, oxygen, or piperazine, which are highly toxic toward several species of parasitic worms, may at the same time be only slightly active against other organisms. In contrast to these, nonelectrolytic anthelminthics must in principle act on different biological objects. From all that is known about the nonspecificity of narcotic action, there is no reason to suspect that any species of parasitic helminth or nonparasitic organism will be insensitive to the action of narcotics.

3. The Antiprotozoal Action of Nonelectrolytes

Besides helminths, other organisms and, in particular, parasitic protozoa inhabit the intestine. They are also found in other hollow viscera communicating with the external environment, for example, in the sex organs. Can we use the principle of nonelectrolytic action in the trial of new antiprotozoal as well as new anthelminthic drugs?

Investigations in this direction were conducted in Lazarev's laboratory by Zaugol'nikov and his collaborators (Zaugol'nikov and Sukhanova, 1952; Karapetyan, 1954; Zaugol'nikov, 1955a, 1955b, 1956). Trichomonads—protozoa belonging to the class Mastigophora—may live in the intestine, the sex organs, and the oral cavity of man. Although the intestinal form of trichomoniasis (<u>Trichomonas intestinalis</u>) may give rise to no symptoms, in carriers and as a complication of bacterial infections trichomoniasis of the sex organs (<u>Tr. vaginalis</u>) is a well-defined nosological entity, responding with difficulty to treatment. Trichomonads are also found in various animals belonging to different systematic groups. Trichomoniasis of the sex organs of cattle is a cause of sterility, and is therefore responsible for much loss of stock. In spite of numerous chemotherapeutic trials, no satisfactory agent has yet been obtained against trichomonads (for a survey of the literature, see Zaugol'nikov, 1956).

Zaugol'nikov and Sukhanova (1952) found that in laboratory conditions 95% of albino mice show intestinal infestation with <u>Trichomonas muris</u>. The most common site of habitation of trichomonads in these animals is the cecum. The suitability of this "model" for trials of new drugs against trichomoniasis has been verified by the assessment of the efficacy of the existing antiprotozoal preparations used in human trichomoniasis against the intestinal trichomoniasis of mice. Carbazone, stovarsol, and — to a lesser degree — yatren, effectively decrease the extent

TABLE 14. Action of Anthelminthics and Benzene against Trichomoniasis (figures from Karapetyan,1954)

Substances	Intensity of infestation (conventional units)	
	in the control group	in the treated group
Hexylresorcinol	3.6	1.2
Thymol	3.6	1.4
Carbon tetrachloride	3.2	0.3
	3.7	0.3
Benzene	3.2	2.0

of the infestation in a group of animals, whereas salol and sulfathiazole, for example, which are ineffective against human trichomoniasis, also have no action on intestinal trichomonads. The activity of carbazone, stovarsol, and of garlic or onion juice against trichomonads in experiments on mice was subsequently confirmed by Karapetyan.

Quantitative indices have been introduced to evaluate the efficacy of chemotherapy: the morbidity index (the percentage of affected mice) and the intensity of infestation, determined by the number of trichomonads visible in a film of cecal contents. Karapetyan used this technique to investigate the action of certain anthelminthics against trichomoniasis. He tested substances for which the value of the coefficient MLD/LC_{50}, according to Zakabunin's figures (Table 13), exceeded unity: hexylresorcinol, thymol, carbon tetrachloride, and benzene. It was previously shown that these substances possess anthelminthic activity. All obviously reduced the intensity of infestation of mice with trichomonads (Table 14).

It was also found that substances for which the value of the coefficient is low, for example, bromural, have no action on trichomonads (Zaugol'nikov, 1956).

We may conclude that the principle and method of selection of anthelminthic drugs with nonelectrolytic action may also be used for the trial of drugs for use against protozoa and trichomonads.

Chapter 4
TRIALS OF NEW ANTHELMINTHIC AND ANTIPROTOZOAL DRUGS

The hypothesis that the mechanism of action of carbon tetrachloride and similar anthelminthic substances is nonelectrolytic has been confirmed by direct experiment. A method of trial of new anthelminthic substances with nonelectrolytic action has been suggested. It has been found that the principle of nonelectrolytic action may be used to test not only anthelminthic drugs, but also drugs against protozoa and, in particular, against trichomonads (Zaugol'-nikov, 1955a, 1955b, 1956; Karapetyan, 1954). The way has thus been prepared for the trial of new anthelminthic and antiprotozoal drugs with nonelectrolytic action.

1. Anthelminthic Drugs

The first step in the trials was the selection of compounds: determination of the coefficient MLD/LC$_{50}$; the second — investigation of the selected compounds in experiments on infested animals. The compounds were selected by the techniques described in the previous chapter: in experiments on nematodes and infusoria. The results of this stage of the work are summarized in Table 15.

Experiments were conducted with hydrocarbons, haloid-substituted hydrocarbons, alcohols, phenols, aldehydes, ketones, ethers, esters, nitro compounds, and urethanes.

Certain compounds naturally had no action on nematodes and paramecia, and others were active only in saturated solution. These compounds were excluded from further investigation. Compounds for which the value of the coefficient MLD/LC$_{50}$ was less than unity also were not investigated. Among the 48 compounds for which the coefficient was greater than unity were several which had previously been tested as anthelminthics. Naphthalene, for example, is a component of many mixed anthelminthic preparations, and it has sometimes been used in the pure form (Oelkers, 1943). Dibenzyl ether, according to Deschiens and Marchal (1945) proved highly effective when tested in cats with oxyuriasis. Diphenylamine has been used successfully for ascariasis in dogs (Guthrie, 1940), but it was later given up, evidently because its deriviative thiodiphenylamine (phenothiazine) proved more effective.

Data concerning the anthelminthic activity of two compounds, hexachlorocyclohexane (hexachlorane) and citral, were published soon after our own researches. Hexachlorocyclohexane was used in small doses in enterobiasis (Brede, 1949). The anthelminthic action of citral was discovered by Zibitsker and Bukhovtseva (1952). These workers used citral to diminish the allergic reactions in patients with ascariasis. To their surprise, besides its antiallergic action, the drug proved to behave as an anthelminthic.

Certain hitherto unstudied compounds characterized by a high coefficient MLD/LC$_{50}$ and therefore promising were tested in experiments on animals. These include: the hexene-hexane and heptene-heptane fractions of synthetic benzine, freon-112, freon-113, several ethers and esters, octanal, and octyl alcohol.

Trials of Compounds in Experiments on Cats Infested with Toxocara mystax and Dipylidium caninum

Method of treatment of toxocariasis. The animals selected were those in which examination of the stools revealed infestation with T. mystax. On the day before treatment, a saline laxative was given through a tube: a 10% solution of magnesium sulfate in a dose of 10 ml/kg body weight. Control experiments showed that this dose of laxative causes the expulsion of not more than 3-5% of helminths of this species infesting cats. The test preparations were administered next morning, also through a tube. Immediately thereafter the laxative was repeated in the previous dose. Expulsion of the helminths from the animals was recorded for 3 days. At the end of this period, the cats were sacrificed, the intestine removed and examined, and the number of specimens of T. mystax remaining was counted.

TABLE 15. Minimal Lethal Doses for Albino Mice by Enteral Administration (MLD), Concentrations Immobilizing 50% of Nematodes or Paramecia (LC$_{50}$), and Coefficients MLD/LC$_{50}$ (Paribok, 1956)

Group	Compound	MLD for mice (in g/kg)	LC$_{50}$ for nematodes (in g/liter)	LC$_{50}$ for paramecia (in g/liter)	$K = \dfrac{\text{MLD}}{\text{LC}_{50}}$
Hydro-carbons	Hexane	15.5	—	None	—
	Hexene-hexane fraction of synthetic benzine	25	—	0.03	833
	Heptene-heptane fraction of syntheticbenzine	5	—	0.012	416
	Iso-octane	—	—	None	—
	Iso-decylene	25	—	None	—
	Shale benzine	—	—	None	—
	Naphthalene	0.428	—	0.0214	20
	Naphthalan oil	—	—	None	—
	Cyclohexane	0.8	—	0.09	8.9
Chlorine-substituted hydro-carbons	Benzyl chloride	0.35	—	0.071	5
	Dipentene chloride	—	—	None	—
	Myrtenyl chloride	—	—	None	—
	1-Chloromethylnaphthalene	1.8	—	None	—
	Hexachlorocyclohexane	0.3-0.6	—	0.06	5-10
	DDT	1.6	—	None	—
Freons	Monochlorodecafluorobutane	5.7	—	0.19	30
	Freon-112	12.2	—	0.013	940
	Freon-113	32.8	—	0.064	390
Alcohols and phenols	Methyl alcohol	10.7	63	—	0.17
	Ethyl alcohol	10.0	43.5	—	0.23
	Isopropyl alcohol	6.0	21	—	0.28
	Isobutyl alcohol	4.0	5.2	—	0.77
	Isoamyl alcohol	2.0	2.5	—	0.80
	Hexyl alcohol	2.5	0.68	—	3.7
	Heptyl alcohol	3.5	0.27	—	12.9
	Secondary octyl alcohol	2.0	0.13	—	15.3
	Benzyl alcohol	—	—	None	—
	Cyclohexanol	0.8	—	0.9	0.9
	Benzhydrol	—	—	None	—
	1,7-Dihydroxynaphthalene	0.4	—	None	—
	2,3-Dihydroxynaphthalene	0.5	—	0.123	3.9
	2,7-Dihydroxynaphthalene	0.4	—	0.34	1.18
Aldehydes	Hexanal	3.5	0.346	—	10.1
	Heptanal	5.0	0.22	—	23
	Octanal	6.0	0.187	—	32
	Citral	3.0	—	0.09	33
	Paraformaldehyde	—	—	None	—
	Benzaldehyde	—	—	None	—
Ketones	Methyl-propyl ketone	2.0	5.2	—	0.38
	Diethyl ketone	2.0	4.03	—	0.49
	Methyl-isobutyl ketone	2.0	2.5	—	0.8
	Dipropyl ketone	2.0	0.88	—	2.27
	Methyl-amyl ketone	2.0	0.78	—	2.56
	Methyl-hexyl ketone	2.0	0.214	—	9.4
	Benzophenone	1.8	0.08	—	22
	Ionone	5.0	0.085	—	59
Simple ethers	Di-isopropyl	2.5	—	0.5	5
	Di-isoamyl	7.5	—	0.03	250

(continued on next page)

TABLE 15 (continued)

Group	Compound	MLD for mice (in g/kg)	LC$_{50}$ for nematodes (in g/liter)	LC$_{50}$ for paramecia (in g/liter)	K = $\dfrac{MLD}{LC_{50}}$
Simple ethers (cont'd)	Dibenzyl	2.9	—	0.029	100
	Methylnaphthyl	—	—	None	—
	Ethylnaphthyl	—	—	None	—
	Naphthylbenzyl	—	—	None	—
	Methylmetacresyl	0.8	—	0.08	10
	Methylorthocresyl	3.0	—	0.06	50
Esters and lactones	Amyl acetate	6	—	1.2	5
	Benzyl acetate	4.5	—	0.45	10
	Phenylethyl acetate	10	—	0.2	50
	Decalyl acetate	0.3	—	0.015	20
	Terpenyl acetate	1.5	—	0.03	50
	Linolyl acetate	12.6	—	0.021	600
	Methylglycol acetate	—	—	None	—
	Ethyl butyrate	23.7	—	2.37	10
	Amyl butyrate	25.8	—	0.086	300
	Amyl valerianate	12	—	0.04	300
	Diethyl ester of isovalerianic acid	—	—	None	—
	Amyl salicylate	4.2	—	0.006	700
	Benzyl salicylate	—	—	None	—
	Isopropyl benzoate	13.0	—	0.065	200
	Ethyl cinnamate	—	—	None	—
	Methyl anthranilate	5.5	—	0.55	10
	Dimethyl fumarate	28.4	—	5.68	5
	Monobutyl ester of glycol	—	—	None	—
	Monoethyl ester of glycol	51	—	51	1
	Ethyl ester of 2-butoxycyclopropane-1--carbonic acid	13.7	—	0.275	50
	Di-isobutyl maleinate	—	—	None	—
	Isohexyl adipinate	—	None	None	—
	Ester of ethylene glycol and iso-oleic acid	—	None	None	—
	Diethylene glycol ester of isovalerianic acid	—	None	—	—
	Butyrolactone	—	—	None	—
Nitro compounds and imines	Diphenylamine	1.6	—	0.0126	127
	Dibenzylamine	0.3	—	0.03	10
	1-Nitropropane	4.9	—	2.42	2
	1-Nitrobutane	2.7	—	0.89	3
	Nitro-alizarin	—	—	None	—
Urethanes	Phenylurethane	—	—	None	—
	Naphthylurethane	—	—	None	—
	Thiourethane	0.3	—	0.06	5
	Amylene carbamate	—	—	None	—
	Diphenyl carbamate	—	—	None	—
	Di-isobutyl carbamate	—	—	None	—
Misc. compounds	Nitryl of adipinic acid	1.9	—	1.98	1
	Phenylhydrazine	—	—	None	—
	Alizarin	—	—	None	—
	Anthraquinone	—	—	None	—

Note: The word "None" denotes substances acting on helminths or paramecia only in saturated solution or having no action whatever on these organisms.

TABLE 16. Treatment of Toxocariasis of Cats with Synthetic Benzine Fractions and Other Hydrocarbons (Paribok, 1953a)

Compound	Dose (g/kg)	Total number of animals	Number of animals		Number of helminths	
			from which helminths were expelled	cured completely	expelled	found in intestine
Hexene-hexane fraction	0.5	4	2	1	6	5
Heptene-heptane fraction	0.3-0.5	4	4	2	15	4
Octene-octane fraction	0.5	4	3	1	21	4
Nonene-nonane fraction	0.5	4	4	3	39	2
Kerosene	0.5	4	0	0	0	—*
Hexadiene-hexene mixture	0.5	4	2	2	8	10

* The cats in this group were not examined post mortem.

Method of treatment of dipylidiasis. When this research was being carried out in Leningrad, the rate of infestation of cats with D. caninum was almost 100%, and absence of infestation was a rare exception. Cats were accordingly used in the experiment without preliminary stool examination. The plan of treatment was as described above; expulsion of helminths was recorded for 2 days. The efficacy of the anthelminthics in dipylidiasis was assessed by comparing the number of helminths found post mortem in the experimental and control animals.

Besides D. caninum, T. mystax was expelled from many animals. Other species of helminths and, in particular, Hydatigera taeniaformis were much less common.

Hydrocarbons. The hexene-hexane and heptene-heptane fractions of synthetic benzine* were tested in experiments on cats infested with T. mystax. Besides these compounds, the anthelminthic action of which could be foreseen from pilot experiments (Table 15), certain higher fractions of synthetic benzine were tested. All these compounds had a marked anthelminthic action. In a series of compounds the efficacy increased with lengthening of the hydrocarbon radical: after administration of the hexene-hexane fraction about 50% of all specimens of T. mystax infesting the animals' intestine was expelled, but after the same dose of the nonene-nonane fraction, 39 of 41 helminths of this species were expelled (Table 16).

TABLE 17. Anthelminthic Activity of Saturated Hydrocarbons in Toxocariasis in Cats (Paribok, 1953a)

Compound	Dose (g/kg)	Total number of animals	Number of animals		Number of helminths	
			from which helminths were expelled	cured completely	expelled	found in intestine
Hexane	0.5	4	4	0	8	9
Heptane	0.5	4	2	2	2	21
Octane	0.5	4	1	0	1	64
Nonane	0.5	4	0	0	0	10

The preparations showed side effects in the form of irritation of the gastrointestinal tract (salivation and vomiting) and slight depression of the central nervous system. The lower fractions gave the most marked side effect, and the octene-octane fraction the least. Administration of the latter caused vomiting in only one cat. The behavior of the remaining animals was normal.

The tested fractions consisted of a mixture of saturated and unsaturated hydrocarbons. In order to discover which part of the fraction is responsible for the anthelminthic activity — the saturated or unsaturated — experiments were carried out with saturated hydrocarbons containing the same number of carbon atoms. The activity of the saturated hydrocarbons was significantly weaker, and moreover, an increase in the length of the hydrocarbon radical in this case led to a decrease rather than an increase in efficacy. Hexane showed the strongest activity; nonane was completely inactive (Table 17).

* The hydrocarbons and hydrocarbon mixtures were supplied for the investigation by D. M. Rudkovskii, head of the All-Union Petrochemical Research Institute Laboratory.

TABLE 18. Anthelminthic Activity of Nonene in Toxocariasis of Cats

Dose (g/kg)	Total number of animals	Number of cats		Number of helminths (T. mystax)	
		from which helminths were expelled	cured completely	expelled	found in intestine
0.5	3	2	2	3	4
0.25	4	3	2	14	12
Control (laxative)	6	1	0	1	33

Note: In this and the subsequent tables the number of helminths (expelled or found in the intestine) refers to the whole group of animals receiving that particular dose.

TABLE 19. Anthelminthic Action of Nonene in Dipylidiasis of Cats

Dose (g/kg)	Total number of cats	Number of animals in which helminths were found post mortem	Number of helminths found in cats post mortem
0.5	9	2	93
0.25	9	2	331
Control 1 (laxative)	9	8	774
Control 2 (untreated)	9	8	over 400

Of the unsaturated hydrocarbons, nonene was tested and proved effective (Tables 18 and 19). Nonene, however, caused severe irritation of the gastrointestinal tract of the animals, and vomiting frequently occurred. Some of the drug was thus wasted and the efficacy of treatment was reduced. This is evidently the reason why nonene was less effective than the nonene-nonane fraction, of which nonene accounted for not more than 25%.

To find out how the anthelminthic activity of the hydrocarbons changes with a further increase in the number of double bonds, experiments were conducted with hexadiene, the molecule of which contains two double bonds. Hexadiene was diluted with hexane in proportions so that the fraction of unsaturated hydrocarbon in the mixture corresponded to that in the hexene-hexane fraction. The two fractions were found to be roughly equally active (Table 16).

It had to be explained why, with an increase in the number of carbon atoms, the anthelminthic activity of a series of synthetic benzine fractions, on the one hand, and the activity of a series of saturated hydrocarbons, on the other hand, should change in opposite directions: an increase in the first case and a decrease in the second. [*] As we mentioned in the second chapter, in a series of nonelectrolytes arranged in order of decreasing solubility in water (i.e., for example, in a homologous series of hydrocarbons), the biological activity increases until a particular member of the series is reached, after which it completely disappears, for the solubility is insufficient for the activity to be exhibited. The increase in anthelminthic efficacy thus requires no special explanation. A sudden disappearance of activity at a certain level would cause no doubt (see p. 7). The situation, however, is quite different; the activity of the saturated hydrocarbons weakens gradually; each member of the series has a weaker action than its predecessor.

The explanation is evidently as follows. In animal experiments the concentration of the drug in the intestine falls continuously after its internal administration because of absorption into the blood stream and subsequent excretion. The concentration of the more soluble, i.e., the more readily absorbed substances, falls more rapidly. This may be judged, for example, by comparing the amount of hexyl- and heptylresorcinol excreted via the kidneys; the absorption of hexylresorcinol amounts to 25%, and that of the less-soluble heptylresorcinol to only 5% of the administered dose. In equal doses, the higher homologs, which are absorbed slowly from the intestine, are active against helminths longer than the lower, so that instead of a sudden disappearance of the effect, it gradually weakens.

The anthelminthic activity of technological products—mixtures of saturated and unsaturated hydrocarbons of different molecular weight—has often been utilized in veterinary and medical helminthological practice. Because of their low activity, however, these substances (benzine, kerosene) are rarely used. It may be seen from Table 16 that the anthelminthic activity of fractions of synthetic benzine is much stronger than that of kerosene (kerosene in a dose of 0.5 g/kg generally does not cause expulsion of helminths).

[*] In experiments on rats, Whitlock (1945) also observed a decrease in the anthelminthic activity of a homologous series of saturated hydrocarbons.

29

TABLE 20. The Activity of Freons in Toxocariasis of Cats (Paribok, 1956)

Compound	Dose (g/kg)	Total number of cats	Number of animals		Number of helminths (T. mystax)	
			from which helminths were expelled	cured completely	expelled	found post mortem
Freon-112	0.1-1.0	14	12	9	38	22
Freon-113	0.5	6	3	0	14	22

TABLE 21. The Activity of Freons in Dipylidiasis of Cats

Compound	Dose (g/kg)	Total number of cats	Number of cats in which helminths were found post mortem	Number of helminths found
Freon-112	1.0	9	1	7
Freon-112	0.5	9	2	117
Freon-113	0.5	9	1	32
Control 1 (laxative)	—	9	8	744
Control 2 (untreated)	—	9	8	over 400

TABLE 22. Anthelminthic Activity of Benzophenone and Ionone in Toxocariasis in Cats (Paribok, 1953b)

Compound	Dose (g/kg)	Total number of cats	Number of cats		Number of helminths (T. mystax)	
			from which helminths were expelled	cured completely	expelled	found post mortem
Benzophenone	0.25	4	4	1	35	11
Ionone	0.5	2	1	0	4	6

Freons. [*] The high value of the coefficient MLD/LC$_{50}$ for freon-112 (difluorotetrachloroethane) and freon-113 (trifluorotrichloroethane) — 940 and 390, respectively — suggested that these freons might have anthelminthic properties. They were accordingly tested in toxocariasis and dipylidiasis of cats. The freons showed marked anthelminthic activity in both infestations (Tables 20 and 21).

Freons are extremely stable and chemically inert. The bond between the atoms of carbon and fluorine is much stronger than the bond with chlorine. Moreover, the appearance of a fluorine atom in the molecule also increases the strength of the bonds between carbon and the other elements. In view of these circumstances, the anthelminthic activity of the freons may be considered to afford further confirmation of the nonelectrolytic mechanism of action of anthelminthic drugs. Because of the chemical inertia of the freons, the suggestion that their action on helminths may have a specific mechanism becomes highly improbable.

Ketones. In the course of trials of new anthelminthics, no systematic investigation of the ketones has yet been undertaken; the activity of some ketones on helminths has been tested only in vivo or on preparations made from helminths. No experiments have been conducted on infested animals.

The results of the preliminary investigations of ketones, given in Table 15, reveal the pattern described in Chapter 3 regarding the changes in the toxic concentrations and lethal doses of nonelectrolytes in homologous series. With an increase in the length of the hydrocarbon radical, the toxicity of ketones toward the nematode Cosmocerca ornata increases continuously: ionone, for example, acts 130 times more strongly on the nematode than methyl-propyl ketone. The toxicity toward higher animals of ketones administered internally changes very little; ionone is actually less toxic than methyl-propyl ketone toward mice. Because of this fact, the value of the coefficient MLD/LC$_{50}$ rises as the hydrocarbon radical lengthens.

Judging by the value of the coefficient MLD/LC$_{50}$, the last two ketones tested (benzophenone and ionone) may exhibit anthelminthic activity. Experiments on cats affected by toxocariasis confirmed this suggestion (Table 22).

[*] The freons were supplied for the investigation by the State Institute of Applied Chemistry.

TABLE 23. Lethal and Therapeutic Doses of Preparations Tested Against Hymenolepidiasis of Albino Mice (Paribok, 1957a)

Preparation	LD_{50} for the mouse (g/kg)	Therapeutic dose (0.2 LD_{50}, g/kg)
Benzophenone	2.0	0.4
Nonene-nonane fraction of synthetic benzine	32.1	6.4
Freon-112	23.5	4.7
Freon-113	32.2	7.2
Ethereal extract of male fern	0.85	0.17
Carbon tetrachloride	4.36	0.87
Tetrachloroethylene	4.00	0.80

Alcohols, aldehydes, ethers, and esters. Cats affected with toxocariasis were used in trials of the anthelminthic activity of octyl alcohol, octanal (Paribok, 1953b), di-isopropyl and dibenzyl ethers, amyl salicylate, linolyl acetate, amyl butyrate, amyl valerianate, and terpenyl acetate (Zakabunin, 1952). All the compounds tested showed some anthelminthic activity: helminths were expelled from some animals after administration of the preparations in doses of 0.25-0.5 g/kg. This activity was much weaker, however, than that of the freons and hydrocarbons. Some compounds (octanal, octyl alcohol) moreover, caused severe irritation of the gastrointestinal tract and made the animals vomit. The weak activity of the esters may be due to hydrolysis of the molecules of these compounds in the alkaline medium of the intestine. During hydrolysis, one molecule of an ester, which has a strong action on helminths outside the body, forms two molecules of weaker narcotics: an alcohol and an acid. These compounds are readily soluble and quickly absorbed, and evidently cannot exert sufficient activity on helminths in the intestine.

Trials of Substances in Hymenolepidiasis of Albino Mice

The activity of substances which had proved effective in the treatment of toxocariasis in cats — the nonene-nonane fraction of synthetic benzine, freon-112, freon-113, and benzophenone (the first three were also effective in dipylidiasis in cats)— was investigated in an experimental cestode infestation: hymenolepidiasis of albino mice. Infestation of albino mice with the dwarf tapeworm (Hymenolepis nana) follows a similar course to hymenolepidiasis in man. After the ova of the tapeworm have entered the intestine, larvae are hatched out (cysticercoids). These pass into the intestinal villi, grow, and compress the blood vessels. The villi necrose and the grown cysticercoids once again enter the lumen of the bowel. Here the adult forms attach themselves to the intestinal wall and begin to liberate ova. The whole developmental cycle of the worm from the moment of infection to the beginning of ovulation takes three weeks. The activity of anthelminthics can be studied on both the cysticercoids, which are the larval stage, and the adult forms.

Technique. The mice were infected by introducing the washings and fragmented helminths obtained from dehelminthization of an affected child into the stomach through a tube. Because of the occurrence of a relative age-immunity (Badalyan, 1955), the experiments were conducted on young animals weighing 9-14 g, which are most susceptible to infection. The stools were examined 20 days after infection for the presence of helminth ova. From the evening before treatment began, the infected animals were changed over to a water-sugar diet, which aided the removal of formed masses from the intestine (Burn et al., 1950).

All the compounds were administered once only, 20-25 days after infection of the animals, i.e., with the intention of acting on the adult stage of the helminths. The nonene-nonane fraction of synthetic benzine and the freons were given undiluted; their volume was made up to 1 ml with water. The remaining substances were injected in the form of a suspension in gum arabic. This suspension was prepared in an electric homogenizer. The dose was 0.2 LD_{50} (Table 23).

Certain known anthelminthics (extract of male fern, tetrachloroethylene, and carbon tetrachloride) were tested for comparison with the new compounds. With one exception, the experiment with each substance was conducted on 30 mice: tetrachloroethylene was given to 25 mice. Two hours after receiving the preparation, the mice were given 1 ml of 6.4% magnesium sulfate solution. After a further 3-5 hours, the animals were sacrificed by decapitation, the intestine was opened throughout its length, and the helminths found there were counted (under the binocular microscope). Animals in which no helminths were found were regarded as cured.

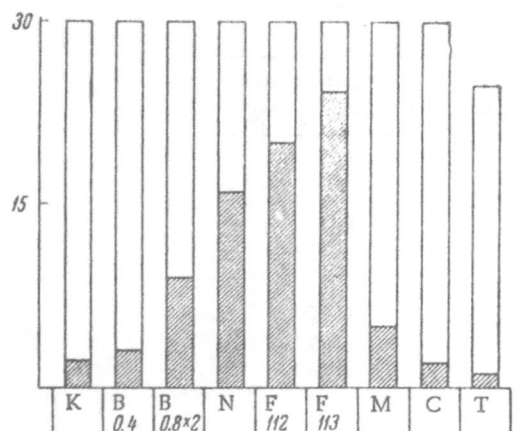

Fig. 8. Results of the treatment of experimental hymenolepidiasis in albino mice. The shaded portion of the columns represents the number of mice cured. K — control; B 0.4 — benzophenone in a dose of 0.4 g/kg; B 0.8 × 2 — benzophenone in a dose of 0.8 g/kg, twice; N — nonene-nonane fraction of synthetic benzine; F-112 — freon-112; F-113 — freon-113; M — extract of male fern; C — carbon tetrachloride; T — tetrachloroethylene.

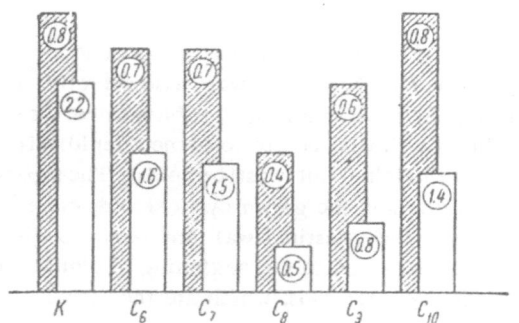

Fig. 9. Action of synthetic benzine fractions against trichomonads. The shaded columns represent the incidence of infestation; the unshaded columns, the intensity of infestation. K — control group; C_6-C_{10} — groups of animals treated with hexene-hexane, heptene-heptane, octene-octane, nonene-nonane, and decene-decane fractions of synthetic benzine, respectively. Figures from Zaugol'nikov (1956).

Results. The new anthelminthic compounds tested in these experiments showed obvious anthelminthic activity in hymenolepidiasis (Fig. 8). Freon-113 was the most effective; 24 of the 30 mice so treated were free from helminths. A much weaker effect was given by administration of extract of male fern, tetrachloroethylene, and carbon tetrachloride. Statistical analysis by the Student — Fisher method showed that the results of the experiments with the freons and the nonene-nonane fraction of synthetic benzine were significant.

Trials undertaken on the basis of the hypothesis of the nonelectrolytic action of anthelminthic drugs thus led to the discovery of a series of compounds having obvious anthelminthic activity in animal experiments: freons 112 and 113, the nonene-nonane fraction of synthetic benzine, and benzophenone. The positive result of the trials confirms the correctness of the original assumptions and the desirability of using the suggested method of investigation of substances in pilot selection experiments. We may note that the same compounds (freons, nonene-nonane fraction of synthetic benzine) exhibited an anthelminthic action in infestations by both nematodes and cestodes. This fact confirms the hypothesis that their anthelminthic activity is nonelectrolytic (nonspecific) in its mechanism.

What are the prospects of the practical application of the results of this research? Firstly, it would be useful to conduct trials of the compounds discovered in ascariasis, hymenolepidiasis, and the teniases, i.e., in infestations caused by helminths from the systematic point of view closely related to the agents of the diseases in the animals in the experiments described above. There is no reason to suppose that these drugs will be effective in infestations by extraintestinal helminths such as, for example, schistosomiasis or the filariases. The blood concentration of the narcotic, when doses tolerated by the host are given, will be insufficient to exert a toxic action on parasites in the blood stream. So far as the helminths infesting the biliary tract are concerned, there is no reason why it should not be possible to treat these infestations with nonelectrolytic anthelminthics. The nonelectrolyte concentration in the venous blood flowing from the intestine is considerably greater than that in the arterial blood (see Chapter 5). It is therefore possible that the concentration of the drug in the biliary tract carried to the liver by the portal venous blood, as a result of excretion in the bile will be sufficient to exert its action on helminths. The likelihood of attacking parasites in the liver would naturally be greater if they were more sensitive to the toxic action of the drug than the helminths inhabiting the intestine.

2. Antiprotozoal Drugs

Karapetyan (1954) investigated the activity of the octene-octane fraction of synthetic benzine against trichomonads in experiments on albino mice infested with intestinal trichomonads. The preparation showed an obvious chemotherapeutic action. As a result of the administration of octene-octane fraction for 2 weeks in a dose of 1.1 ml/10 g body weight, the mice were completely cured of the infestation.

Further studies of the action of nonelectrolytes against trichomonads were made by Zaugol'nikov (1955a, 1955b, 1956). Among the synthetic benzine fractions, consisting of mixtures of saturated and unsaturated hydrocarbons, the octene-octane fraction showed greatest activity against trichomoniasis of mice (Fig. 9). In contrast to the anthelminthic activity of hydrocarbons, the saturated hydrocarbons were no less active against trichomonads than the unsaturated. In the series of saturated hydrocarbons the greatest activity also was shown by octane.

The octene-octane fraction of synthetic benzine was subsequently tested as the preparation "synoctane" in the treatment of human trichomoniasis and of analogous diseases of domestic animals.

Chapter 5

SIDE-EFFECTS OF NEW CHEMOTHERAPEUTIC SUBSTANCES
WITH NONELECTROLYTIC ACTION

The antibiotics penicillin, streptomycin, tetracycline, and others are examples of chemotherapeutic substances with a well-marked selectivity of action. The toxicity of antibiotics toward sensitive microorganisms is hundreds of times greater than their toxicity toward the higher animals (Spector, 1957). Despite this fact, antibiotic therapy is attended by several side-effects, limiting their potential application. Far more serious side-effects occur during the use of certain anthelminthic and antiprotozoal preparations with selective toxicity toward parasites. For example, after the administration of santonin, xanthopsia (yellow vision) is, as a rule, observed, and during the treatment of teniases with male fern preparations irritation of the mucous membrane of the gastrointestinal tract and several manifestations affecting the central nervous system may take place. Various, and often severe, side-effects may accompany the use of antimalarial preparations.

What is to be expected in this respect from anthelminthic and antiprotozoal substances with nonelectrolytic action? As we showed in Chapter 2, in principle these drugs are more toxic to the host than the parasites, and they exert their selective action on the parasites as a result of the temporary selective accumulation at the site of infestation. It is well known that anthelminthic substances with nonelectrolytic action at present used in medical and veterinary helminthological practice cause side-effects of varying severity, and that some of them, if a slight overdose is given, may give rise to considerable toxic manifestations. For instance, the main obstacle to the widespread use of carbon tetrachloride is its high toxicity. The danger thus may arise that the side-effects of the new preparations discovered as a result of our researches may be so severe that their use is generally precluded.

From the pharmacological point of view the anthelminthic drugs with nonelectrolytic action are narcotics. Besides their resorptive action, narcotics also have a local action: they cause, for example, irritation of mucous membranes. Certain narcotics, mainly belonging to the group of haloid-substituted hydrocarbons, damage the parenchymatous organs, especially the liver. Finally, it must be ascertained whether the chemotherapeutic use of anthelminthic substances with nonelectrolytic action is attended by any resorptive narcotic action on the host — depression of the central nervous system.

So far as drugs intended for local application against trichomonads are concerned, it is their local action on mucous membranes that is of greatest concern.

In this chapter we describe the side-effects associated with the following anthelminthic and antiprotozoal preparations: freon-112, freon-113, the nonene-nonane fraction of synthetic benzine, benzophenone, and synoctane (the octene-octane fraction of synthetic benzine).

1. The Action of Anthelminthic Preparations on the Intestinal Epithelium

Besides helminths, the intestinal wall and the epithelium of the gastrointestinal tract are exposed to the action of anthelminthics introduced into the bowel. The intestinal epithelium is bathed by the same solution of poison as the helminths. The sensitivity of the epithelial cells to narcotics is of the same order as that of intestinal helminths (Makarov, 1938). Hence, it follows that during administration of anthelminthic preparations with nonelectrolytic action the intestinal epithelium apparently must be affected to no less a degree than the intestinal helminths. Is this in fact so?

Information regarding the action of anthelminthics on the intestinal epithelium is available, although it is scanty. Large doses of carbon tetrachloride, greatly in excess of the therapeutic dose, are known to cause excretion of mucus from animals (Shul'ts, 1931). After taking carbon tetrachloride internally, patients observed a feeling of warmth in the region of the stomach (Pod'yapol'skaya and Kapustin, 1958). No histological changes in the mucous membrane of the intestine after administration of carbon tetrachloride are described. No details are available of the effect of tetrachloroethylene or of other drugs, including those investigated in the present research, on the intestinal epithelium. Hexylresorcinol occupies a special place in regard to its action on the epithelium of the gastrointestinal tract. Resorcinol is a keratolytic substance and causes marked irritation of the mucous membrane. The higher homologs of resorcinol and, in particular, heptylresorcinol, also possess an irritant action, although less marked. According to Lamson, Brown, and Ward (1935a), who conducted experiments on dogs, to Maplestone and Chopra (1934) — on cats, and to Anderson et al. (1931) and Vol'f (1948) — on rabbits, hexylresorcinol causes a series of changes in the gastric mucosa: necrosis of the epithelium, and hemorrhages into the submucosal and mucosal layers. These lesions were found after administration of toxic or lethal doses of hexylresorcinol to patients. It must be stressed that the injurious action of hexylresorcinol was detected mainly in the mucous membrane of the stomach. Only Vol'f, who gave rabbits 5 therapeutic doses of hexylresorcinol (0.15 g/kg), observed necrosis of the epithelial cells in the proximal part of the intestine, together with focal hemorrhages and edema of the submucosa. No lesions were observed after administration of therapeutic doses of hexylresorcinol.

Adequate information on the injurious action of the drug on the intestinal epithelium is thus available for only one anthelminthic substance with nonelectrolytic action: hexylresorcinol. The other drugs evidently do not injure the epithelium. This conclusion is very encouraging for the therapeutic application of these substances. It is difficult, however, to agree with the hypothesis that their activity is nonelectrolytic in nature, bearing in mind the closely similar (roughly equal) sensitivity of the epithelium and the helminths to narcotics.

It might be supposed, for example, that the injury to the epithelium is slight and, moreover, reversible, so that it cannot be detected by the usual histological treatment of fixed tissues. There are, however, more sensitive methods of detection of the initial stages of cell injury, for example, by the method of vital staining. Many dyes, especially neutral red, do not stain the cytoplasm and nucleus of uninjured cells. The dyes collect in the cytoplasm in the form of granules. This is a manifestation of the defensive reaction of the cell to the action of a foreign substance. After the cell is injured, the character of its staining changes radically. The dye stains the cytoplasm diffusely; it also stains the nucleus, which normally is invisible. These changes in the staining properties of the cell after injury have been investigated in detail by Nasonov and Aleksandrov (1940). This group of changes and, in particular, the changes in the ability of the cell to be stained by basic and acid dyes, or paranecrosis, is found in association with injuries less severe than those associated with the subsequent gross histological changes.

We used the vital staining technique to investigate the action of the following anthelminthics on the intestinal epithelium: carbon tetrachloride, tetrachloroethylene, hexylresorcinol, freon-113, the nonene-nonane fraction of synthetic benzine, and benzophenone. The first three compounds are widely used anthelminthics; the mechanism of the action has been proved to be nonelectrolytic (Chapter 2). The anthelminthic action of the other three substances was discovered on the basis of the hypothesis of the nonelectrolytic action of anthelminthics, and is described in the previous chapters.

The substances were introduced into the stomach or rectum of albino mice in amounts equal to half the lethal dose ($LD_{50}/2$). The mice received no food during the 8 hours before administration of the preparation. Carbon tetrachloride and tetrachloroethylene were given in emulsion form, hexylresorcinol and benzophenone as suspensions, and freon-113 and the nonene-nonane fraction in undiluted form, the volume being made up to 2 ml with Ringer's solution. After different, predetermined intervals, the animals were given 3 ml of a 0.005% solution of neutral red, diluted in Ringer's solution without soda: 1 ml into the stomach and 2 ml into the rectum. After staining of the intestine for 15 minutes, the mice were decapitated and the intestine removed; sections of the duodenum, ileum, and large intestine were cut and examined under the microscope. Each substance was administered to not less than eight mice: to four, into the stomach, and to the rest, into the rectum. In the experiments with each substance, the dye was given after 15 minutes, 30 minutes, 1 hour, and 12 hours (once only to each animal).

In no case were signs of injury of the intestinal epithelium observed throughout its extent after administration of carbon tetrachloride, hexylresorcinol, the nonene-nonane fraction of synthetic benzine, freon-113, or benzophenone, whether into the stomach or into the rectum, and whatever the duration of their action (from 15 minutes to 12 hours). The dye was collected into granules, the cytoplasm was unstained, and the nuclei remained invisible. Only in two of the 32 experiments with tetrachloroethylene were paranecrotic changes observed at the apices of the villi: staining of the nuclei and diffuse staining of the cytoplasm. These were discovered in mice in a state of severe depression after receiving large doses ($LD_{50}/2$) of the preparations. A normal, uninjured state of the intestinal epithelium is thus typical of the action of the anthelminthic drugs which we tested.

The suspicion may arise that the anthelminthics are retained in the stomach or, if administered rectally, in the lower parts of the intestine. Passage of the liquid substances into the intestine (the experiments with carbon

TABLE 24. The Action of Anthelminthics on the Protozoa Trichomonas muris in the Intestine of the Albino Mouse

Substance	Concentration of suspension (in %)	Mode of administration	Duration of action							
			15 min				30 min			
			D	J	I	L	D	J	I	L
Hexyl-resorcinol	0.5	Stomach	+	+	+	+				
		Rectum	−	−	+	+				
Carbon tetrachloride	8	Stomach	+	+	+	+				
		Rectum	+	+	+	+				
Freon-113	Undiluted	Stomach	+	−	−	−				
		Rectum	−	−	−	−				
Nonene-nonane fraction of synthetic benzine	Undiluted	Stomach	+	+	−	−				
Benzophenone	2	Stomach	−	−	−	−	+	+	+	+
		Rectum	−	−	−	−	+	+	−	−

Note: The "−" sign denotes that the protozoa are motile; the "+" denotes that the protozoa are nonmotile. D — duodenum; J — jejunum; I — ileum; L — large intestine.

TABLE 25. Action of Anthelminthics on the Epithelium of Isolated Segments of the Intestine of the Albino Mouse

Substance	Concentration (in %)	Number of mice	Duration of action (min)					
			3	5	10	15	20	25
Hexylresorcinol	0.17 and 0.5	3	+	+	+	+		
Carbon tetrachloride	8	3		+	+	+		
Tetrachloroethylene	2 and 8	5		±	+	+		
Freon-113	100	2			±	±		
Nonene-nonane fraction of synthetic benzine	100	8				−	−	±
Benzophenone	2	4		+	+	±	±	
Control (Ringer's solution)	−	22	−	−	−	−	−	−

Note: The "+" sign denotes a paranecrotic character of staining; the "−" sign denotes normal (granular) staining.

tetrachloride, tetrachloroethylene, and nonene-nonane fraction) was confirmed by coloring them before administration, using the dye Sudan II. In this case, drops of the injected substance stained the characteristic orange color were found in the intestine of the mice, and often a colored drop was seen in contact with an uninjured epithelial cell containing neutral red granules. The crystalline substances hexylresorcinol and benzophenone could be seen in the intestine without special staining.

Further and no less convincing proof of the passage of the anthelminthic drugs into the intestine was given by the state of the protozoa Trichomonas muris inhabiting that region. In control mice these protozoa were always found in every part of the intestine, and they were actively motile. Their state in the intestine of the experimental animals is shown in Table 24. After the action of each of the tested substances, areas of the intestine could be found (usually near the site of administration of the preparation) where the protozoa were immobile. We may remember that in the experiments on the treatment of hymenolepidiasis (Chapter 4) the administration of much smaller doses of the preparations (0.2 LD_{50} percent) led to expulsion of the helminths from the intestine.

The anthelminthic substances with nonelectrolytic action thus reach the intestine, where they exert a toxic action on the helminths and parasites present, without injuring the intestinal epithelium. The explanation of this phenomenon is evidently that the conditions of action of the anthelminthics on the intestinal epithelium and the helminths are different. The helminths are completely immersed in the solution of the poison in the intestinal contents; in contrast to this, the epithelial cells have only one surface facing the lumen of the intestine. Their opposite surface is in contact with the deeper layers of the mucous membrane, with their rich blood supply. The conditions of elimination of absorbed poison from the epithelial cells are naturally more favorable than the conditions of its

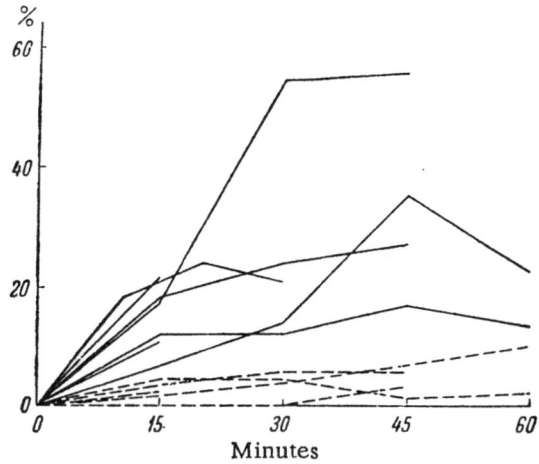

%

Fig. 10. Absorption of tetrachloroethylene from the intestine. The concentration of the compound in the venous blood flowing from the intestine and in the arterial blood is expressed in percent of its concentration in the solution passing through the lumen of the bowel (the concentration of the solution is taken as 100%). Continuous line — venous blood; broken line — arterial blood; each line corresponds to an experiment on one animal.

elimination from the helminths, so that the mean concentration of poison in the epithelial cell must be less than in the body of the helminths. In other words, there is a falling gradient of concentration from the lumen of the bowel to the blood vessels supplying its wall.

In order to verify this statement, experiments were carried out in which the concentration of tetrachloroethylene was estimated simultaneously in the intestinal fluid and the blood flowing from the intestine. Because of the small size of the blood vessels in the mouse, samples of blood flowing from the intestine could not be taken, and the experiments were accordingly performed on cats.

Tracheotomy was performed under ether anesthesia. After changing over to intratracheal anesthesia, laparotomy was performed. A loop of bowel was brought out of the wound and placed in a kidney dish containing warm Ringer's solution. A glass cannula was inserted into one of the intestinal veins toward the mesenteric vein. A glass tube was tied into the lumen of the bowel for perfusion purposes. The arteries and veins supplying the other parts of the intestine were ligated, and only those vessels supplying blood to the exteriorized loop of bowel were preserved. A cannula was introduced into the common carotid artery. Perfusion of the intestine (through its lumen) with a saturated solution of tetrachloroethylene in Ringer's solution, warmed to 38°, then began. Samples of perfusion fluid and of blood from the mesenteric vein and carotid artery were taken periodically. The concentration of tetrachloroethylene in the perfusion fluid was determined by direct photometry in ultraviolet light, using the SF-4 spectrophotometer (Paribok, 1957a). The tetrachloroethylene in the blood was determined after extraction with hexane.

The experiments showed that the concentration of tetrachloroethylene in the intestinal perfusion fluid is 3 to 4 times higher than its concentration in the blood flowing from the intestine (Fig. 10). Consequently, the suggestion that a fall of concentration of tetrachloroethylene takes place from the intestinal fluid to the blood vessels was confirmed.

In the work of Lasarus and Rogers (1951), cited above, simultaneous determinations were made of the anthelminthic drug phenothiazine, labeled with sulfur (S^{35}), in the body of the helminths, and in the blood and epithelium of the host. The phenothiazine concentration in the epithelium in experiments on chicks was slightly higher than in the blood, but much less than in the body of the helminths. In experiments on rats, the concentration of phenothiazine in the epithelium was even lower than in the blood (expressed in terms of dry weight of tissue).

The presence of a concentration gradient and of a lower concentration of an anthelminthic substance in the epithelium than in the body of the helminths is thus not in doubt. This being so, it may be considered that the abolition of this gradient must lead to injury of the intestinal epithelium, during the action of concentrations of anthelminthic substances harmless to it in normal conditions. This was verified in experiments on isolated segments of intestine.

The small intestine was removed from a decapitated white mouse which had been starved for 8-12 hours before the experiment. Pieces of intestine, opened longitudinally, were placed in vessels containing anthelminthic substances (in the form of suspensions or in the undiluted state) in the concentrations used in the experiments on the intact animals. After intervals of 5, 10, 15, 20, and 25 minutes, the pieces were transferred to a 0.05% solution of neutral red in soda-free Ringer's solution for 10 minutes. After staining, the pieces were rinsed and examined under the microscope.

The anthelminthic substances acting on the isolated pieces of intestine cause injury to the intestinal epithelium. Paranecrotic changes are found: diffuse staining of the cytoplasm and staining of the nuclei (Table 25). The degree of injury varied. Hexylresorcinol had the strongest action; the nonene-nonane fraction of synthetic benzine caused the least injury. In the experiments with all these substances, a certain duration of exposure could be found at which paranecrotic changes took place in the epithelial cells. In the control experiments the staining of the epithelium was invariably granular in character.

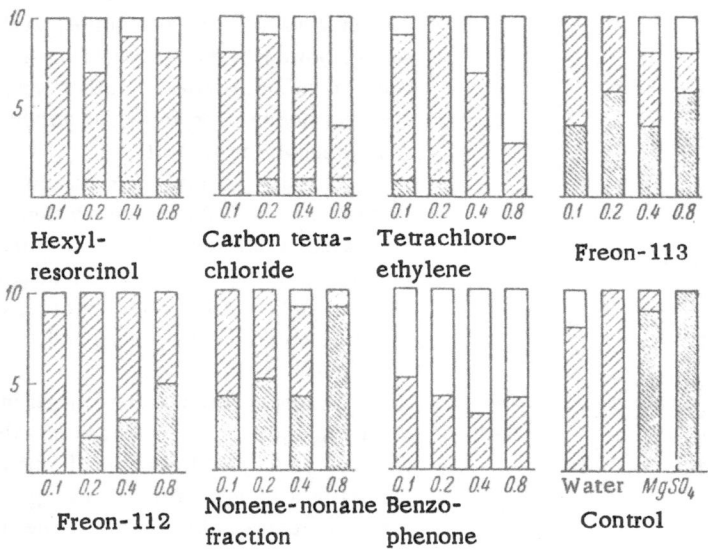

Fig. 11. The effect of anthelminthic drugs on intestinal function. The figures beneath the columns denote doses in fractions of LD$_{50}$; height of the column — number of animals. Shaded part of the column — number of animals showing diarrhea; lightly shaded part — number of animals with normal intestinal function; unshaded part — number of animals showing constipation.

Paranecrotic changes thus appear very quickly (in the experiments with hexylresorcinol after less than 5 minutes) in the epithelium of isolated pieces of the intestine in response to the action of anthelminthics. It will be recalled that the same substances in the same concentrations caused no injury in experiments on intact animals, even when the experiment was of much longer duration. These results are in agreement with the previous findings, and accord fully with the suggested explanation of the absence of paranecrotic changes in the epithelial cells of the intestine after introduction of anthelminthic substances into the gastrointestinal tract of animals.

2. The Effect of Anthelminthic Substances on Intestinal Function

In the course of treatment of intestinal helminthiases, immediately after the anthelminthic drugs the patients usually receive laxatives in order to remove the unabsorbed portion of the drug and also the helminths, which have become incapable of remaining in the intestine. It would be advantageous, of course, if the anthelminthic substances themselves were laxatives. Such drugs do exist: they include, for example, kamala, which is now rarely used. Conversely, it would be undesirable and inconvenient to use anthelminthics with a constipating action.

When the side-effects of new anthelminthic drugs are being evaluated, it must therefore be established whether they have a laxative or a constipating action, or whether they have no effect on the intestinal function.

The effect of some anthelminthic drugs used in current medical practice, and also of new drugs, on the intestinal function may be investigated by Fuhner's method (Sargin, 1936).

Albino mice are starved for 4 hours before the experiment, and the drug is then administered by means of a gastric tube, either in undiluted form or as a suspension in gum arabic. Immediately after the drug, 0.5 ml of a suspension of ink in water is administered. Ink is used because it permits clearer registration of the laxative effect. The mice are kept on sheets of paper under bell-jars, and the results of the experiment are recorded after 4 hours by means of an arbitrary scale.

The experiments showed that hexylresorcinol, carbon tetrachloride, and tetrachloroethylene in doses of 0.1 to 0.2 LD$_{50}$ do not affect the intestinal function (Fig. 11). After receiving larger doses (0.4-0.8 LD$_{50}$), some animals develop constipation, evidently as a result of general depression. Freon-112, freon-113, and nonene-nonane fraction caused looseness of the stools. Benzophenone, even in small doses, caused constipation. The laxative action of the freons and the nonene-nonane fraction of synthetic benzine may be explained by the fact that, because of their low toxicity, these substances were given in relatively large doses. Being poorly absorbed, they caused a considerable increase in the bulk of the intestinal contents.

3. The Action of Anthelminthics on the Liver

The side-effect of anthelminthic drugs on the liver has been estimated by the hexenal test (Wenzel and Gibson, 1951). Injury to the liver, resection of that organ, or partial restriction of the blood flow through the liver (Eck's fistula) cause a great increase in the duration of hexenal and of thiopental narcosis (Shideman et al., 1947).

The experiment was conducted as follows. Hexenal was injected intraperitoneally into male rats, and the time from injection of hexenal to waking was measured. During the following days the animals received the test substances, after which the hexenal test was repeated.

The test substances were administered to the rats through a gastric tube in doses of 0.2 LD_{50} (see Table 22 for the mouse). The duration of hexenal narcosis increased considerably in the rats which received carbon tetrachloride (Fig. 12). This finding agrees with the results of Wenzel and Gibson, and indicates severe liver damage. In the experiments with freon-112, freon-113, and the nonene-nonane fraction of synthetic benzine, the duration of narcosis was not significantly lengthened. In contrast to the other substances, benzophenone shortened the duration of narcosis. According to Sokolova, working in our laboratory, benzophenone also shortens the duration of medinal narcosis, presumably by lowering the sensitivity of the central nervous system to the narcotic.

The new anthelminthic substances freon-112, freon-113, nonene-nonane fraction of synthetic benzine, and benzophenone, unlike carbon tetrachloride, do not, therefore, cause disturbances of liver function. In the case of freon-112, this result was confirmed by histological investigation of the liver of the rats, which was undertaken by our colleague, O. I. Smirnova.

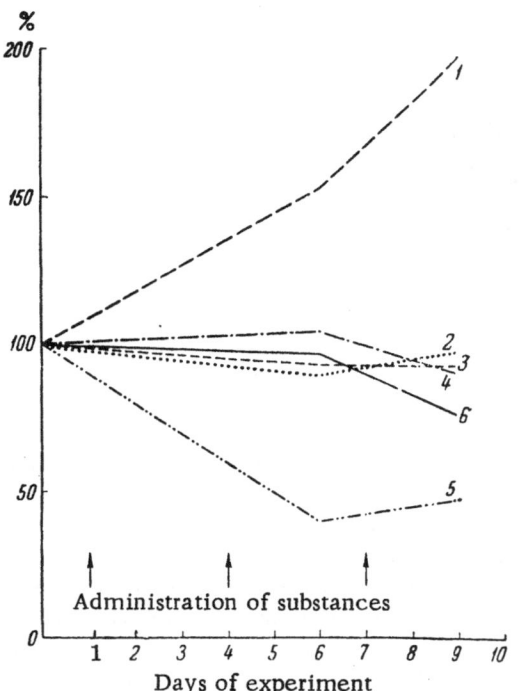

Fig. 12. The effect of anthelminthics on the duration of hexenal narcosis in rats: 1) carbon tetrachloride; 2) nonene-nonane fraction of synthetic benzine; 3) freon-112; 4) freon-113; 5) benzophenone; 6) control group.

4. The Action of Anthelminthics on the Central Nervous System

Depression of the central nervous system takes place during treatment with carbon tetrachloride and tetrachloroethylene. It takes the form of slight manifestations of intoxication.

The action of the new anthelminthics on the central nervous system was studied in experiments on dogs in which motor-food conditioned reflexes had been established by the method of free choice of feeding bowl. The following indices were recorded: the presence of an orienting reaction, the duration of the latent period of the reflex, the presence and the correctness of the conditioned reaction, the reaction to the differential stimulus, and the unconditioned reaction. Experiments were carried out on two dogs with stable conditioned reflexes and well-established differentiation. The test substances were administered through a gastric tube or fed with a small piece of meat. The doses used (in terms of body weight) were those which, in experiments on cats, had a marked anthelminthic action (Chapter 4). The conditioned reflex activity of the dogs was investigated the day before the experiment, 30 minutes after administration of the preparation, and thereafter for two days.

The experiments showed that benzophenone (0.25 g/kg), freon-112 (1.0 g/kg), and freon-113 do not interfere with the conditioned reflex activity of dogs.

5. The Action of Drugs Active Against Trichomoniasis on the Mucous Membrane

In experiments on rabbits, Zaugol'nikov (1956) studied the local action of synthetic benzine fractions possessing antiprotozoal activity and used against trichomoniasis. The substances were instilled into the conjunctival sac.

Within 24 hours of the instillation of hexene-hexane fraction of synthetic benzine, erythema of the conjunctiva and encrustations on the lid margins were observed. No changes were seen in the conjunctiva after a single instillation of the higher fractions of synthetic benzine — heptene-heptane and decene-decane. These fractions caused no irritation after four instillations. We may recall that in experiments on cats the higher synthetic benzine fractions also exhibited an insignificant irritant action (Chapter 4).

Chapter 6

TRIALS OF NEW CHEMOTHERAPEUTIC DRUGS
WITH NONELECTROLYTIC ACTION
IN MEDICAL AND VETERINARY PRACTICE

1. The Action of Freon-113 in Ascariasis

The action of freon-113 in ascariasis has been tested in certain Leningrad hospitals.[*] For therapeutic use, the preparation was called "triftol." As a first step it was established that, in a dose of up to 12 g, the preparation causes no pathological manifestations or unpleasant sensations in healthy subjects, with the exception of a feeling of fullness in the stomach and occasional eructation of wind.

On the night before treatment the patient was given a cleansing enema and a saline laxative (25-30 g magnesium sulfate). The preparation was given in gelatin capsules to the patients on an empty stomach, and this was followed by a repetition of the saline laxative in the same dose. Observations were made on 35 patients. Depending on the method of treatment, they could be divided into six groups. The first group of patients received one dose of 9 g triftol, followed 20 minutes later by a laxative. In 5 (of the total number of 13) patients, ascarids were expelled as a result of treatment. Complete disinfestation from helminths was achieved, however, in only one patient. The second group of patients received triftol in a dose of 12 g. The laxative was given 20 minutes later. Expulsion of ascarids was observed in 3 of the 5 patients. Because of the shortness of their stay in the hospital it was impossible to verify that disinfestation was complete by subsequent stool analysis.

The patients of the third and fourth groups received triftol in doses of 9 g and 12 g, and a laxative 2 hours later. Ascarids were expelled from only 3 patients. Finally, when triftol was administered after a dose of sodium bicarbonate (to ensure that the drug passed more rapidly into the intestine by opening the pylorus) — group 5 — and by reducing the dose to 6 g (group 6), expulsion of ascarids was not observed. The most effective method was thus to give a dose of 12 g and to follow this with a laxative after 20 minutes.

2. Trials of Freon-113 in Hymenolepidiasis

The action of freon-113 (triftol) in hymenolepidiasis was tested clinically by the Research Institute of Malaria and Medical Parasitology of the Ministry of Health of the Turkmenian SSR (Ashkhabad).[**] Eleven patients (7 adults and 4 children) were treated. Many of the patients were infested only to a mild degree; not more than 1-3 ova were counted in one field of vision. The children were more severely infested. Before receiving triftol, three patients had been treated with male fern preparations, but without good results.

Each patient was given a laxative on the night before treatment; next morning a cleansing enema was given, and then the triftol: adults received 15-20 g and children 4-11 g. A saline laxative was given 20 minutes after administration of the triftol. Expulsion of helminths was recorded for 3 days. Before the beginning and after the end of treatment, a full blood count and analysis of the urine and feces were carried out on all patients. The feces were again analyzed for helminth ova 10 days after the end of treatment.

Because of the localization of the larvae (cysticercoids) in the substance of the villi, the preparation, as might have been anticipated, had no action on the larval form of the helminths. In accordance with the general principle, treatment was therefore given in the form of several courses, in order to act upon the adult specimens entering the lumen of the intestine in the early stages. The second course was given 10 days after the first, and the third 10 days after the second. On the first day of the course of treatment the patient received 15-20 g triftol, and on the second day 10-15 g, followed by a laxative 20 minutes later. Four patients received three courses of treatment. Two were

---

[*] The investigation was carried out by Dr. É. G. Blik.
[**] The investigation was carried out by Dr. Mizgireva, under the direction of G. A. Pravikov and F. F. Soprunov.

TABLE 26. Anthelminthic Action of Freon-113 (Triftol) in Human Hymenolepidiasis (according to Mizgireva, Pravikov, and Soprunov)

Patient	Number of courses	Results of treatment (ova of Hymenolepis nana)
K-a	3	Not found
K-t	3	Not found
K-va	3	Found
T-o	3	Found
S-a	2	Not found
I-n	2	Found
Z-v	1	Found
Z-a	1	Not found
A-v	1	Not found
F-t	1	Not found
Z-a	1	Found

completely cured (Table 26). One of two patients was cured after two courses of treatment. The results of treatment of 5 patients who received one course (in 3 cases analysis showed absence of ova of the dwarf tapeworm) are regarded reservedly by these workers. They consider that parasites in the larval stage, insusceptible to the action of the preparation, could still remain in the patients' intestines. Nevertheless, it is obvious that triftol had an appreciable effect in human hymenolepidiasis. In 6 of 11 patients, adult specimens of Hymenolepis nana were expelled from the intestine as a result of treatment.

After taking triftol, the patients noticed vertigo, nausea, and eructation of wind with the odor of triftol. These manifestations were very slight and transient; they passed off after 15-20 minutes. Blood examination revealed a slight increase in the hemoglobin concentration as a result of loss of water from repeated administration

of the laxative. No pathological changes were detected in the heart, liver, kidneys, or other internal organs.

3. Trials of Freon-112 and Freon-113 in Ascariasis

These trials were conducted at the Pushkin Stock-Rearing Laboratory.[*]

Control necropsies on adult cockerels of the "Leghorn," "New Hampshire," and "First of May" breeds from the laboratory farm showed a high incidence of infestation with Ascaris galli. The cockerels were divided into groups so that each group contained equal numbers of birds kept under identical conditions before the experiment. The control cockerels were untreated; the experimental cockerels received freon-112 (3 g/kg) or freon-113 (2 and 3 g/kg). Both preparations were introduced into the gizzard through a special tube. Throughout the experiment the birds were kept on the same diet. To evaluate the results of treatment, cockerels were sacrificed 2 days after receiving the preparations, and the ascarids in the intestine were counted.

Of the 16 control (untreated) cockerels, 14 were infested. The number of ascarids found in these birds was 47. Of the 16 birds receiving freon-112, ascarids were found in only two. At post-mortem examination of the 15 cockerels receiving freon-113, helminths were found in three, and the other 12 birds were free from infestation.

Freon-112 and freon-113 were thus shown to be highly effective anthelminthics in ascariasis. Observations on the birds after administration of the preparations showed no abnormality. The meat of birds killed 48 hours after treatment had no unusual smell or taste. We may mention that freons can easily be given into the gizzard of the birds by means of a forced-feeding machine as used in poultry farms.

4. The Use of Freon-112 in Fascioliasis in Sheep

The efficacy of freon-112 in fascioliasis was tested by N. V. Demidov of the Academician K. I. Skryabin All-Union Institute of Helminthology (Demidov, 1955, 1957). In a preliminary experiment, freon-112 was given to two rabbits and 5 sheep infested with liver fluke (Fasciola hepatica) in doses of 0.3 and 0.6 g/kg, and proved therapeutically 100% effective, with no side-effects. Freon-112 was next tested on a wider scale in commercial conditions. The compound was given to sheep in doses of 10-20 ml (16-32 g). Four sheep were sacrificed after 24 hours. One fluke was found in the bile ducts of one of these sheep, and 3 flukes in another. The other 2 sheep were absolutely free from flukes. In another experiment 15 sheep were treated with freon-112 for infestation with Fasciola hepatica. The compound was given in doses of 20-25 ml (32-40 g) by injection through the abdominal wall, directly into the paunch. The stools were reexamined 11 days later. This showed that all the sheep were completely cured of fascioliasis.

Trials at the Meat Combine, undertaken without preliminary selection of infested animals, also showed that freon-112 is highly effective in fascioliasis.

In Demidov's experiments only a few sheep reacted to the administration of freon-112 by transient excitation; in most animals there were no side-effects.

In recent years (Demidov, 1955, 1957) the scale of trial of freon-112 has been extended considerably. This compound was used in the treatment of 1112 sheep in 2 flocks in which the incidence of infestation was 17 and 48%,

---

[*]These investigations were conducted by V. P. Paribok and S. I. Bogolyubskii.

respectively. Freon was injected into the paunch in a dose of 8-10 ml (13-16 g) with, as a rule, no change in the feeding routine. Subsequent analyses showed that the efficacy of treatment of fascioliasis under these circumstances is 100%. Demidov cites the results of these investigations as evidence that freon-112 is harmless in practice and a highly effective preparation for the treatment of fascioliasis.

5. Treatment of Trichomonas Vaginitis by the Octene-Octane Fraction of Synthetic Benzine

The results obtained by Zaugol'nikov and Karapetyan from their experiments on the treatment of trichomonas infestation of mice provided the basis for trials of the most effective substance — the octene-octane fraction of synthetic benzine— in clinical conditions. The preparation used in clinical trials was called "synoctane." Timeskova (1955) treated 43 women suffering from trichomonas vaginitis with synoctane. Eighteen of these patients had been treated previously with stovarsol, the antibiotic "binan," streptocide, and other preparations, but without result. Vaginal smears from all the patients showed the presence of Trichomonas vaginalis.

The patients were treated by insertion of tampons soaked in a 50% solution of synoctane in peach oil into the vagina. Solutions of this concentration, in contrast to the more highly concentrated, did not irritate the mucous membrane. The course of treatment lasted 4-6 days on the average. As a rule, good results were observed within a few days of the application of synoctane. The volume of discharge was reduced, and the distressing pruritis and sensation of burning ceased. The hyperemia of the mucous membrane was also considerably diminished. Control examinations of smears for 2 months during and after treatment showed absence of trichomonads in 65% of patients.

In cases where vaginal smears again showed the presence of trichomonads, a further course of treatment was given. This, however, proved of little value. In view of lack of knowledge of the epidemiology of trichomoniasis, it was uncertain whether this was the result of reinfection or of recurrence of the original disease.

6. The Use of the Octene-Octane Fraction of Synthetic Benzine in Trichomoniasis of Cattle

Trichomoniasis of cattle (trichomonas vaginitis, and a combination of trichomonas vaginitis and endometritis) is a cause of infertility in cattle and is responsible for much wastage in stock breeding. In view of the similarity between the epidemiology and pathogenesis of trichomoniasis in cattle and the corresponding disease in man, Zaugol'-nikov suggested the use of synoctane for treatment of this infestation.

Sokolov (1955) used synoctane in 50 cows with infertility due to trichomoniasis. The preparation was introduced on tampons for 6-8 hours, and the course of treatment lasted 6 days. In the chronic disease, undiluted synoctane was used, and in the acute form a 75% solution of synoctane in peach oil. The clinical manifestations of vaginitis subsided after 3-4 procedures, and after 5-6 applications of synoctane, the inflammatory phenomena cleared up completely in most patients. As a result of the application of synoctane, 9 animals suffering from acute trichomonas vaginitis were cured. A cure was also effected in 27 cows with a chronic form of vaginitis (of a total number of 31 animals treated), although after 3 weeks the disease recurred in 4 of these cows. Of 10 cows with catarrhal or suppurative endometritis, 8 were cured (the information about the other 2 animals was not available).

The results of the trial of new anthelminthic and antiprotozoal substances with nonelectrolytic action thus show that they have a definite therapeutic effect. In certain infestations (ascariasis, trichomoniasis in man) the action of the preparations is weaker than the action of those in current use in medical practice. In human hymenolepidiasis, and also in ascariasis in birds, the preparations are roughly equally effective to the anthelminthics now available. Finally, the efficacy of freon-112 in fascioliasis is much higher than that of all other preparations hitherto tested against this infestation. Good results have also been obtained from the treatment of trichomoniasis in cattle with synoctane.

The trials of chemotherapeutic substances with nonelectrolytic action, the results of which are described in this and the preceding chapters, are based on Lazarev's (1944a, 1944b) hypothesis that the action of certain anthelminthics is nonelectrolytic in nature. The results of these trials have proved successful. The hypothesis has thus been verified and has acquired the character of a scientific forecast.

Chapter 7

THE PRINCIPLE OF NONELECTROLYTIC ACTION IN CHEMOTHERAPY

1. The Use of Substances with Nonelectrolytic Action in Extraintestinal Infestations

Chemotherapeutic effects based on nonelectrolytic action may be of importance in the treatment of infestations of the bowel and the sex organs, i.e., of hollow viscera communicating with the external environment. This condition — the communication between the organ and the environment — enables a high concentration of the substance to be produced within the organ, so that it can exert a toxic action on the parasite. Is this condition essential? If so, how can the anthelminthic action of carbon tetrachloride and freon-112 (Chapter 6) in helminthiases of the liver (fascioliasis) be explained? In infestations of the liver the action does not take place in the intestine, but in the bile ducts and the secretory biliary capillaries where the liver flukes live. It is impossible for the substance to pass from the duodenum into the bile ducts against the flow of bile. It must therefore be admitted that freon-112 and other drugs acting on liver flukes reach the habitat of the parasites after absorption from the intestine, i.e., via the portal vein. The chemotherapeutic effect in this case, in contrast to the effect in intestinal helminthiases, thus takes place after the substance has entered the blood stream and has circulated through some of the blood vessels. The substance does not act on the parasite at the point where it is administered, but at a point to which it is conveyed by the blood.

Before concluding from the foregoing remarks that nonelectrolytic activity may take place without direct communication between the organ in which the parasites live and the external environment, we must establish that, in this case, the action of freon-112 and carbon tetrachloride is nonelectrolytic. This problem can be solved by comparing the toxic thermodynamic concentrations (according to Ferguson — see Chapter 2) of freon-112 and carbon tetrachloride with the concentrations of substances with known nonelectrolytic (narcotic) action, for example, alcohols. This shows that the thermodynamic concentration of carbon tetrachloride causing immobilization of liver flukes is not less, and the concentration of freon-112 is actually greater than, the thermodynamic toxic concentrations of iso-butyl and iso-amyl alcohols for this particular test object (Table 27).

Hence, it follows that the toxic action of carbon tetrachloride and of freon-112 on the liver fluke is not a specific effect; it is a typical nonelectrolytic action. The chemotherapeutic action of the cellular narcosis type (nonelectrolytic action) may thus be manifested in an organ to which the substance is conveyed by the blood stream, and it is not confined to organs communicating directly with the external environment.

As we have pointed out above, the concentration of an anthelminthic substance in the blood flowing from the intestine is only one-half to one-third that of the concentration within the lumen of the intestine (Fig. 11). From this point of view, the action of freon-112 and carbon tetrachloride on the liver fluke may be explained by making one of the following assumptions. On the one hand, it may be supposed that freon-112 and carbon tetrachloride are concentrated in the liver, and are therefore present in the bile in a higher concentration than in the blood in the portal vein. In this case, it would be easy to account for their possible action on the flukes by postulating that these parasites are at least as sensitive as intestinal helminths to anthelminthic drugs. On the other hand, it may be suggested that liver flukes are more sensitive to these drugs — that they die in the presence of lower concentrations than, for example, the nematodes inhabiting the intestine.

Experiments showed that freon-112 satisfies the second assumption. The toxic concentration of freon for Fasciola hepatica is 100 mg/liter, whereas for Toxocara mystax the corresponding concentration is more than 300 mg per liter. Hence, it follows that the new drugs, with nonelectrolytic action, attain their chemotherapeutic effect on liver helminths largely, if not entirely, because the latter are more sensitive to the action of narcotics.

Other helminths, for example, the cat fluke (Opisthorchis felineus), may also infest the liver. Freon-112 causes death of this helminth in the same concentration as the liver fluke, 100 mg/liter. Although the two parasites are

TABLE 27. The Toxic Action of Nonelectrolytes on _Fasciola hepatica_

Substance	Solubility in water, in mg/liter (S)	Concentration immobilizing 50% of flukes, in mg/liter (LC_{50})	Thermodynamic concentration $\dfrac{LC_{50}}{S}$ 100%
Isobutyl alcohol	100,000	7700	7.7
Iso-amyl alcohol	27,000	4000	14
Carbon tetrachloride	800	89	11
Freon-112	250	100	40

equally sensitive in vitro, freon-112 proved ineffective in opisthorchiasis (experiments of Plotnikov and Vinnikov). Why is there this difference between the results in vitro and in vivo? Demidov obtained good results in fascioliasis in sheep. The unsuccessful treatment of opisthorchiasis was given to cats. The marked difference in the results in the two forms of infestation may therefore be related to differences in the fate of freon in the two species of animal, the parasites of which are equally sensitive in vitro to freon-112. Another explanation, however, is more likely. Infestation with the cat fluke causes more severe reactions on the part of the liver parenchyma and the epithelium of the bile ducts than infestation with liver fluke. In opisthorchiasis the parasites are usually surrounded by muco-purulent fluid. This may make contact between the parasites and the anthelminthic drug difficult, and thereby weaken the action of the latter.

Let us examine whether the chemotherapeutic action of nonelectrolytes may be utilized in cases of infestation of organs other than the intestine, genital tract, and liver with parasites.

For such an action to be possible, at least one of the two conditions mentioned above must be satisfied: either the concentration of the drug at the habitat of the parasites must be increased, or the parasite must be more sensitive to the narcotic than is the "weakest link" — the central nervous system of the host. The organ in which concentration of many foreign substances takes place is the kidney. Certain anthelminthics, for example, the alkyl resorcinols,are concentrated in the urine. With this in view, it may be suggested that the principle of nonelectrolytic action might be used in the treatment of helminthic infestations of the kidneys.

An example of such a parasite is the giant kidney worm Dioctophyme renale, which inhabits the renal pelvis of dogs.

Substances with nonelectrolytic action, as we have shown above, may be used in the chemotherapy of helminthiasis and certain protozoal infestations. Can the principle of nonelectrolytic action be expected to prove successful in the chemotherapy of bacterial infections? This is very doubtful, because bacteria are much less sensitive to narcotics than protozoa and helminths. We may recall that the attempts made during the 1920's to use hexylresorcinol as a urinary and intestinal antiseptic proved unsuccessful. The use of substances of this type in the treatment of virus infections is still less likely to be successful. The situation may change radically if a chemotherapeutic substance is found with both a nonelectrolytic and a specific action, i.e., if, because of a suitable combination of physicochemical properties, the drug can be concentrated preferentially at the site of infestation, and at the same time exert a specific action on the agent causing the disease.

2. The Combined Use of Drugs with Nonelectrolytic and Specific Activity

The combined use of certain anthelminthics, as in the case of other chemotherapeutic preparations, has frequently made the treatment more effective. The value of combining drugs with nonelectrolytic action with specific remedies is exemplified by the combined action of hexylresorcinol and santonin, and also of santonin and freon-113. The chemotherapeutic effect of treatment of cats affected by toxocariasis with combinations of santonin and hexylresorcinol or santonin and freon-113 is far superior to that which might be anticipated from simple summation (see Table 28).

It is important to realize that, besides synergism between the anthelminthics when used in combination, relating antagonism may also take place between their toxic action on the host animal (Paribok, 1951, 1954).

One such combined prescription has proved effective and has been used in medical helminthology (Kamalova and Pipiya, 1953; Egnaryan, 1955). Good results have also been obtained in the treatment of taeniarhynchiasis by a full dose of carbon tetrachloride together with a reduced dose of a male fern preparation. When using this method of treatment, Malikov (1936) observed expulsion of helminths in 100% of cases, whereas many patients remained uncured after treatment with these substances separately.

TABLE 28. The Combined Administration of Anthelminthics in Toxocariasis of Cats

Preparations	Dose (g/kg)	Number of cats	Number of helminths expelled	Number of helminths found at autopsy	Proportion of helminths expelled (%)
Santonin	0.05	4	8	21	28
Hexylresorcinol	0.05	4	4	12	25
Freon-113	0.5	4	13	13	50
Santonin	0.025	4	23	1	96
Hexylresorcinol	0.025				
Santonin	0.05	4	26	0	100
Hexylresorcinol	0.05				
Santonin	0.025	4	25	8	76
Freon-113	0.25				
Hexylresorcinol	0.025	4	21	6	75
Freon-113	0.25				

Combined treatement with anthelminthic drugs may even be justified even if its efficacy is not thereby increased, when its toxicity is appreciably diminished as a result of the lowered dose of each constituent. Kovalev (1955) gives an example of this type. The treatment of taeniarhynchiasis by extract of male fern in conjunction with mepacrine, like the treatment by extract of male fern alone, was successful in only half the patients. The incidence of side-effects, however, was lowered from 66 to 9.5% when the combined method of treatment was used.

The combination of chemotherapeutic substances with nonelectrolytic action with specific remedies may lead to the discovery of more effective methods of treatment not only of intestinal helminthiases, but also of extraintestinal infestations, such as protozoal infestations of the bile ducts, which are highly resistant to the action of available preparations.

3. The Combined Use of Several Substances with Nonelectrolytic Action

May it be desirable to combine two or more chemotherapeutic agents with nonelectrolytic action? By combining narcotics, summation of their effects is obtained. This would seem to dispel doubts about the value of such a combination, were it not for the following circumstance. Nonelectrolytic effects may result from the action of quite large concentrations of narcotics, constituting a high proportion of the concentration of the saturated solution. The gain in strength of the toxic action on the pathogenic agent as a result of summation of the narcotic effects of two or three substances when used in combined form would be "neutralized" if, by dissolving additional substances, the solubility of each constituent in water was decreased, and the concentration of the components of such a mixed preparation was thereby lowered. To give an example, let us assume that the solubility of one component in water is 100 mg%, and that of another is 50 mg%, but when both are dissolved together they "interfere" with each other so that their solubility falls to 50 and 25 mg%, respectively. If simple summation of the action of these substances takes place, no advantage will result from their combined administration. Conversely, an obvious gain will result if the upper limits of solubility of the two substances when dissolved together are 80 and 40 mg%, respectively.

Both variants of relationship between nonelectrolytes may, in fact, be found when they are dissolved together (Paribok, 1956). In Fig. 13 we show the solubility of certain nonelectrolytes in water: thymol (T), naphthalene (N), benzophenone (B), and coumarin (C) when dissolved separately and together in water. The solubility of each substance in the absence of others, irrespective of its absolute value, is taken as 100%. It will be apparent that in combinations of, for example, thymol and coumarin or thymol and benzophenone, the solubility of each of these substances is considerably reduced, but in combinations of thymol and naphthalene, or coumarin and naphthalene, and in mixtures of three substances (excluding water) — thymol + coumarin + benzophenone, and thymol + coumarin + naphthalene— the solubility falls only slightly.

These results suggest that, even if simple summation of nonelectrolytic effects is the only factor considered, the combination of several anthelminthic or antiprotozoal drugs with nonelectrolytic action may give a stronger effect than the administration of the same drugs separately. An example of this type of advantageous combination is that of hexylresorcinol and freon-113 (Paribok, 1951). The anthelminthic action of these compounds when given together to cats affected by toxocariasis was stronger than that obtained by giving twice the dose of each separately.

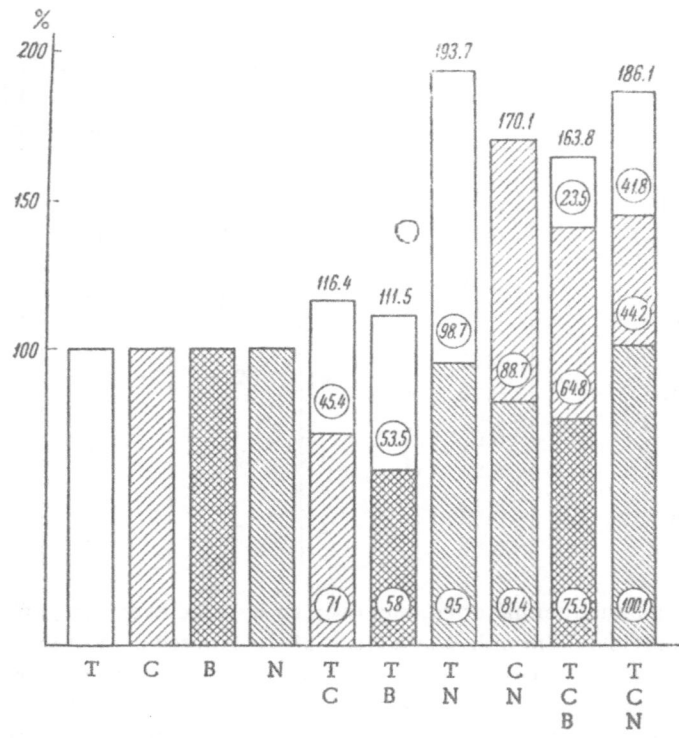

Fig. 13. Solubility of nonelectrolytes in water. For explanation and legend, see text.

4. The Principle of Nonelectrolytic Action and Trials of Specifically Active Chemotherapeutic Substances

The ideal course of chemotherapeutic trials is usually as follows. The metabolism of the parasitic organisms is studied. Its qualitative and quantitative differences from the metabolism of the host are established. Substances are tested for their ability to depress the metabolism of the parasite without affecting or, at least, affecting to a lesser degree, the metabolism of the host.

No objections can be raised, in principle, against this ideal method of trial. Strangely enough, however, it has rarely produced positive results. Albert (1953) made a detailed examination of the conduct of chemotherapeutic trials, and could cite only two successful examples undertaken in accordance with this principle: the introduction of para-aminosalicylic acid (active against tuberculosis) and of phenylpantothenone (active against malaria). One further example could be added to these: the discovery of the anthelminthic action of oxygen against ascarids (Kravets, 1951). The high toxicity of oxygen against ascarids in the adult stage naturally led to the trial of oxygen in ascariasis, in view of its strong toxic action on anaerobes and, in particular, on the anaerobic microflora.

Another more widespread and successful principle of trial of chemotherapeutic substances is that, on the basis of extensive pilot tests, a class of substances having the desired effect (although weak) is discovered, after which substances with the highest possible effect are produced by modification of the chemical structure. This principle has been applied many times to the trial of anthelminthic substances. As examples we may cite tests of the anthelminthic properties of haloid-substituted hydrocarbons(Hall, 1921; Hall et al., 1918, 1925, 1929), alkyl-substituted hydroxybenzene compounds (Lamson et al., 1935a, 1935c), or piperazine derivatives (Hewitt et al., 1947).

Because experiments on helminth-infested animals require a relatively high expenditure of materials and time, much of the work when this method is used is carried out on helminths isolated from the host, i.e., in vitro. Many of the substances tested usually prove toxic toward the helminths, depressing their spontaneous movements or electrically-induced contractions (Baldwin, 1948; Krotov, 1953). At this stage of the trials it is very important to discover the nature of the toxic action of the substance on the parasite. Firstly, it must be ascertained whether the action is <u>specific</u>, i.e., due to a chemical reaction between the substance and some substance in the body of the parasite, or nonspecific (<u>nonelectrolytic</u>).

During the selection of substances by the results of experiments on parasites in vitro, there is thus every reason to use some method which will determine the nature of the effect (narcotic or specific), such as Ferguson's method (see Chapter 2). This enables attention to be concentrated in the future on substances which act specifically, and it may provide the basis for subsequent chemical modifications carried out for the purpose of increasing activity.

5. The Principle of Selective Accumulation

The successes of chemotherapy during more than fifty years have consolidated very securely the place of the principle of selective toxicity, and have led to its spread from medicine to another field of active influencing of nature, that of agriculture (the use of insecticides and herbicides). In fact, the temptation to use this principle is very great! If the metabolism of the pathogenic organism can be suppressed, there is no need to determine accurately the situation of the parasite in its habitat, for example, in the patient's body. Simply by saturating the patient with antibiotics or with the chemotherapeutic agent in an adequate concentration, it is certain that the pathogenic agent will be injured,for the "aiming" of the chemotherapeutic substance at the target of the pathogenic agent was assured before the treatment started; in fact,during the period of research and therapeutic trial.

Besides the good results of the use of this principle, certain essential shortcomings and miscalculations have materialized. It has been found, for example, that interference with biocenosis (the coexistence of organisms inhabiting a given medium, such as, for example, the parasitocenosis of a sick person or animal) may lead to the suppression of some species sensitive to the chemotherapeutic agent by others which are insensitive. An example of such an unfavorable modification of the composition of a parasitocenosis is the candidomycoses — fungus infections arising after the administration of large doses of antibiotics, especially of the broad-spectrum type, as a result of the suppression by the antibiotic of the growth of microorganisms antagonistic to the fungus. In order to overcome this handicap, further specialization of action (increase in the selectivity of action) must be sought, and attempts must be made to obtain greater selectivity of accumulation of the drug at the site of infestation. The treatment of helminthiases and protozoal infestations with chemotherapeutic preparations acting nonelectrolytically is an extreme expression of the principle of selective accumulation, for the effect in this case is due entirely to accumulation of the drug, which may actually be less toxic to the pathogenic agent than to the host. Since an adequate chemotherapeutic effect can result from the application of this one principle alone, it is reasonable to suppose that by a suitable combination of specific action and selective accumulation much more effective chemotherapeutic preparations may be obtained.

BIBLIOGRAPHY

A. Soviet Literature

Albert, E. 1953. Selective Toxicity [Russian translation]. Izd. IL, Moscow.

Badalyan, A. L. 1955. "The age resistance of albino mice to the human dwarf tapeworm." Trudy Inst. Malyarii i Med. Parazitol. Arm. SSR, No. 6, 116.

Baskakov, V. P., Panova, L. G., and Matskevich, V. Yu. 1944. "The results of trials of kerosene in ascariasis,strongyloidiasis, trichonematosis, and oxyuriasis of horses." Veterinariya, 8-9, 18.

Brede, G. D. 1949. "Vermexane, a preparation of gamma-hexachlorocyclohexane, as an anthelminthic." Progress in Therapeutic Preparations, No. 6, p. 9. Moscow.

Davtyan, É. A. 1937. "Experimental treatment of fascioliasis of cattle with hexachloroethane." Trudy Arm. Nauch.-Issled. Veter.-Zootekh. Inst. Narkomzema Arm. SSR, No. 2, 39.

Davtyan, É. A. 1940. "Results of large-scale use of hexachloroethane for fascioliasis of cattle and sheep in the Armenian SSR." Trudy Arm. Nauch.-Issled. Veter.-Zootekh. Inst. Narkomzema Arm. SSR, No. 3, 46.

Demidov, N. V. 1955. "Difluorotetrachloroethane and male fern extract for fascioliasis in sheep." Veterinariya,4,29.

Demidov, N. V. 1957. "Methods of control of fascioliasis in animals." Veterinariya, 10, 33.

Éfendiev, M. É. 1947. "Anthelminthic substances in oriental medicine." Izvest. Akad. Nauk Azer. SSR 5, 1, 23.

Egnaryan, V. O. 1955. "The treatment of ascariasis with santonin, hexylresorcinol and a combination of these preparations." Trudy Inst. Malyarii i Med. Parazitol. Arm. SSR, No. 6, 123.

Ehrlich, P. 1907. "Chemotherapeutic researches into trypanosomiasis." Material on Chemotherapy [Russian translation]. St. Petersburg, pp. 84-120.

El'manov, I. V. 1929. "Carbon tetrachloride in the treatment of fascioliasis in sheep." Collected Works of Veterinary Students from October, 1927 to April, 1928, 1, 1, 82.

Il'inskii, N. I., and Palimpsestov, M. A. 1929. "Carbon tetrachloride as a substance for treatment of fascioliasis of cattle." Vestnik Sov. Vet., 15, 369.

Kadenatsii, A. N. 1947. "Kerosene as an anthelminthic in nematodiases of horses." Veterinariya, 3, 20.

Kamalov, N. G., and Tavlalishvili, Ts. V. 1951. "Treatment of ankylostomiasis and ascariasis with tetrachloroethylene." Med. Parazitol. 20, 3, 26.

Kamalova, A. G., and Pipiya, S. S. 1953. "The combined method of treatment of ascariasis." Med. Parazitol. 22, 5, 404.

Karapetyan, A. E. 1954. Experimental Chemotherapy of the Lambliases and Trichomoniases. Leningrad.

Kovalev, N. E. 1953. Pavlov's Physiological Surgery in the Experimental Therapy of Opisthorchiasis. Moscow.

Kovalev, N. E. 1955. "Experimental treatment of taeniarhynchiasis with male fern combined with mepacrine during mass dehelminthization." Med. Parazitol. 24, 2, 106.

Kravets, N. P. 1951. "Oxygen as an anthelminthic." Med. Parazitol. 20, 2, 122.

Kravets, N. P. 1953. The Oxygen Therapy of Ascariasis. Stanislav.

Krotov, A. I. 1953. "Studies of ascariasis therapy. Report 1. The method of study of reactions of ascarids to chemotherapeutic preparations in vitro." Med. Parazitol., 5, 387.

Krotov, A. I. 1958. "Theoretical basis of the experimental therapy of helminthiases." Trudy Moskovsk. Vet. Akad. 27, 146.

Lazarev, N. V. 1940. The Narcotics. Leningrad.

Lazarev, N. V. 1941. The Biological Action of Gases Under Pressure. Leningrad.

Lazarev, N. V. 1944a. "The correlation between the physicochemical properties of nonelectrolytes and their biological importance." Uspekhi Sovremennoi Biol. 17, 3, 250.

Lazarev, N. V. 1944b. The Nonelectrolytes. Their Biological, Physical, and Chemical Classification. Leningrad.

Lazarev, N. V. (edited by). 1954. Harmful Substances in Industry, Vol. 1. Leningrad.

Lazarev, N. V. 1958. General Information on Narcotics and Narcosis. Leningrad.

Lazarev, N. V., Lyublina, E. I., and Madorskaya, R. Ya. 1948. "The narcotic action of xenon." Fiziol. Zhur. USSR 34, 1, 131.

Machul'skii, S. N. 1938. "The use of Soviet tetrachloroethylene for dehelminthization of dogs." Sovet. Veter. 21, 11, 53.

Machul'skii, S. N. 1941. "Dehelminthization of dogs with Soviet tetrachloroethylene." Trudy Buryat-Mongol'sk. Zoovet. Inst., No. 2, 111.

Makarov, P. V. 1938. "The problem of general and cellular narcosis." Arkh. Anat., Gistol. i Émbriol. 19 1, 5.

Malikov, M. A. 1936. "Taenia saginata and dehelminthization by means of soda, carbon tetrachloride, and extract of male fern." Transactions of the First Congress of the Azerbaijan Medical Society, pp. 313-319.

Nasonov, D. N. 1959. The Local Reaction of the Protoplasm and Spreading Excitation. Moscow-Leningrad.

Nasonov, D. N., and Aleksandrov, V. Ya. 1940. The Reaction of Living Matter to External Influences. Moscow-Leningrad.

Paribok, V. P. 1945. "The relationship between the adhesion properties and narcotic action of nonelectrolytes." Scientific Papers of Students at the Higher Naval Medical School, Naval Medical Academy, No. 5. Leningrad.

Paribok, V. P. 1951. "The combined action of santonin and hexylresorcinol." Med. Parazitol. 20, 6, 554.

Paribok, V. P. 1952. "The principle of trial of anthelminthics with nonspecific action." Med. Parazitol. 21, 5, 417.

Paribok, V. P. 1953a. "The anthelminthic action of saturated and unsaturated hydrocarbons." Med. Parazitol. 22, 3, 248.

Paribok, V. P. 1953b. "The anthelminthic action of aldehydes, ketones, and alcohols." Med. Parazitol. 22, 5, 295.

Paribok, V. P. 1954. The Pharmacology of Anthelminthics. Leningrad.

Paribok V. P. 1955. "The anthelminthics with nonelectrolytic action." Transactions of Scientific Conferences of the Naval Medical Academy, 1, pp. 7-21.

Paribok, V. P. 1956. Anthelminthics with Nonelectrolytic Action. Leningrad.

Paribok, V. P. 1957a. "Comparison of the toxicity of anthelminthic substances to helminths and to the host." Farmakol. i Toksikol. 6, 62.

Paribok, V. P. 1957b. "The toxicity of nonelectrolytic poisons and of some anthelminthics to nematodes." Farmakol. i Toksikol., 4, 74.

Perikhanyan, A. I., and Zorabyan, L. I. 1948. "The treatment of human fascioliasis with hexachloroethane." Klin. Med. 26, 11, 66.

Petrov, A. M., Dzhavadov, M. K., and Gaibov, A. D. 1935. "Experimental trial of tetrachloroethylene in ascariasis and ankylostomiasis of dogs." Trudy Azerb. Nauch.-Issled. Vet. Inst., 2, 53.

Plotnikov, N. N. 1941. "The treatment of opisthorchiasis of cats with hexachloroethane." Doklady Akad. Nauk SSSR 31, 5, 514.

Plotnikov, N. N., and Zerchaninov, L. K. 1932. "The biology of Opisthorchis felineus (Rivolta, 1884) and the treatment of opisthorchiasis." Med. Parazitol. 1, 3-4, 130.

Pod'yapol'skaya, V. P. 1945. "Advances in the treatment of teniases." Med. Parazitol. 14, 2, 79.

Pod'yapol'skaya, V. P., and Kapustin, V. F. 1958. Helminthic Diseases of Man. Moscow.

Potemkina, V. V. 1945. "Experimental therapy of fascioliasis in cattle with hexachloroethane." Veterinariya, 4-5, 26.

Pukhov, V. I. 1932. "The treatment of helminthic infestations (nematodiases) of fowls." Transactions of the North Caucasian Research Veterinary Prophylactic Institute, No. 1, pp. 156-169. Rostov-on-Don.

Sargin, K. D. 1936. The Biological Evaluation of Therapeutic Substances. Moscow.

Selivanov, A. A. 1948. "Treatment of neo-ascariasis of calves." Veterinariya, 1, 26.

Shul'ts, R. S. 1931. Carbon Tetrachloride in Veterinary Helminthological Practice. Moscow.

Shul'ts, R. S. 1933. "The treatment of helminthiases, its mode of development and its present state." Med. Parazitol. 2, 3, 117.

Shul'ts, R. S., and Davtyan, É. A. 1934. "Is tetrachloroethylene suitable as an anthelminthic in fascioliasis." Khimiko-farmatsev. Promysh., 3, 44.

Shul'ts, R. S., and Sutyagin, V. S. 1934. "The treatment of trematodiases in ducks with carbon tetrachloride, tetrachloroethylene and male fern extract." Trudy Vsesoyuzn. Vet.-Zootekh. Inst. im. Zakavkazskoi Feder. 1, 1, 71.

Shul'ts, R. S., and Shikhobalova, N. P. 1934. "In vitro studies of anthelminthics." Med. Parazitol. 3, 6, 528.

Sokolov, N. I. 1955. "The use of synoctane in trichomoniasis in cattle." Transactions of Scientific Conferences of the Naval Medical Academy, 1, pp. 31-33.

Sutyagin, V. S. 1941. "The treatment of ascariasis in cats with tetrachloroethylene." Trudy Erevansk. Vet.-Zootekh. Inst. im. Zakavkazskoi Feder., 5, 164.

Timeskova, G. V. 1955. "The treatment of trichomonas vaginitis with synoctane." Transactions of Scientific Conferences of the Naval Medical Academy, 1, 28-30.

Tuaev, S. M. 1936. "The treatment of enterobiasis with carbon tetrachloride." Med. Parazitol. 5, 5, 814.

Tuaev, S. M. 1954. Enterobiasis and its Treatment by Carbon Tetrachloride. Baku.

Varlakov, M. N. 1939. "Studies of the action of certain anthelminthics on earthworms and Ascaris suilla." Med. Parazitol. 8, 2, 299.

Velichkin, P. A., and Khrapov, G. S. 1946. "Studies of the anthelminthic properties of kerosene in strongyloidiases and para-ascariasis of horses." Vet.-Zootech. Bulletin No. 1 (September), pp. 40-42. Rostov-on-Don.

Velichkin, P. A., and Khrapov, G. S. 1947. "Studies of the anthelminthic properties of kerosene in strongyloidiasis and para-ascariasis of horses." Veterinariya, 3, 20.

Vol'f, N. I. 1948. Clinical Features of Ascariasis and its Treatment with Hexylresorcinol. Sverdlovsk.

Woolley, D. W. 1954. Antimetabolites [Russian translation]. Moscow.

Zakabunin, N. R. 1949. "The method of trial of anthelminthics." Scientific Papers of Students of Faculty 3 of the Naval Medical Academy, No. 6, pp. 129-133.

Zakabunin, N. R. 1952. "The anthelminthic action of ethers and esters." Trudy 9-i Nauch. Konf. Slushatelei Voenno-Morsk. Med. Akad., 98-102.

Zaugol'nikov, S. D. 1955a. "The role of the nonelectrolytic (narcotic) effect in the control of protozoal diseases." Voenno-Morsk. Med. Akad. Mat. Nauch. Konf, 1, 22.

Zaugol'nikov, S. D. 1955b. "The activity of aliphatic hydrocarbons against trichomonads." Farmakol. i Toksikol. 18, 1, 38.

Zaugol'nikov, S. D. 1956. Research in the Field of the Experimental Therapy of Protozoal Diseases. Leningrad.

Zaugol'nikov, S. D., and Sukhanova, K. M. 1952. "The methods of experimental chemotherapy of the trichomoniases." Trudy 4 Nauch. Sessii VMMA, 39 412.

Zenaishvili, O. P. 1951. "The treatment of teniases with Soviet carbon tetrachloride." Byull. Nauch.-Issled. Inst. Malyarii i Med. Parazitol. im. Virsaladze, 2, 46.

Zibitsker, D. E., and Bukhovtseva, A. D. 1952. "The use of citral in the treatment of ascariasis." Med. Parazitol. 21, 1, 81.

B. Non-Soviet Literature

Anderson, H. H., David, N. A., and Leake, C. D. 1931. "Oral toxicity of certain alkyl resorcinols in guinea pigs and rabbits." Proc. Soc. Exp. Biol. Med. 28, 609-612.

Baldwin, E. 1948. "Study of antihelminthic potency in relation to chemical constitution." Brit. J. Pharmacol. 3, 6, 91-107.

Bennet. 1885. Cited by Boas, J., 1889.

Biyal, N. 1948. "Ueber die Wirkung des Reinbenzins auf die Darmparasiten und seine Folgen. Schweiz. Med. Wochenschr. 78, 23, 571-572.

Blair, H. E. 1949. "Vermiplex, a new anthelminthic for dogs." North American Veterinarian 30, 5, 306-309; abstr. see: Helm. Abstr. 18, 2, 103a.

Boas, J. 1889. "Neure Bandwurmmittel und Curen." Deutsch. Med. Wochenschr. 15, 18-19.

Burn, J. H., Finney, D. J., and Goodwin, L. G. 1950. Biological Standardization. London.

Cawston, F. G. 1945. "Chloroform in the treatment of worms." Clin. J. 74, 5, 191-192.

Deschiens, R., and Marchal, G. 1945. "Sur les propriétés anthelmintiques des oxydes et du benzoate de benzyle." Comptes Rendu de la soc. Biol. 139, 7-8, 351-353.

Duguid, A. M. E., and Heathcote, R. St. A. 1950. "Actions of drugs in vitro on cestodes: anthelminthics. Archiv. Int. Pharmacodyn. 82, 301-330.

Enzie, F. D. 1947. "The anthelminthic action of toluene in dogs." Proc. Helm. Soc. Wash. 14, 1, 34-35.

Enzie, F. D. and Colglasier, M. L. 1953. "Toluene (methylbenzene) for intestinal nematodes in dogs and cats." Veterinary Medicine 46, 6, 325-328.

Faure, L. 1940. "Traitement des helmintes equines par le pétrole." Ann. Parasit. Humaine et comp. 17, 6, 590-592; abstr. see: Helm. Abstr. 9, 1, 59.

Ferguson, J. 1939. "Use of chemical potentials as indices of toxicity." Proc. Roy. Soc. London., Ser. B., 127, 367-404.

Gieron, Z. 1954. "Benzina jako srodek przeciwczerwiowy." Przegl. lekar. 10, 6, 190-192.

Guthrie, J. E. 1940. "Preliminary observations on the efficacy of diphenylamine for removal of in.estinal nematodes from pigs." Proc. Helm. Soc. Wash. 7, 2, 84-85.

Hall, M. C. 1919. "Studies on anthelminthics. III. Chloroform as an anthelminthic." J. Amer. Vet. Med. Assoc. 55, 652.

Hall, M. C. 1921. "The use of carbon tetrachloride for the removal of hookworms." J. Amer. Med. Assoc. 77, 1641.

Hall, M. C., and Augustine, D. L. 1929. "Some investigations of anthelminthics by egg and worm count method." Amer. J. Hyg. 9, 584-628.

Hall, M. C., and Foster, W. D. 1918. "Efficacy of some anthelminthics." J. Agric. Res. 12, 7, 397-417.

Hall, M. C., and Shillinger, J. E. 1925. "Tetrachloroethylene, a new anthelminthic." Amer. J. Trop. Med. 5, 229-237.

Hewitt, R. J., Kushner, S., Stewart, White, E., Wallace, W. S., and Subbarow, J. 1947. "Experimental chemotherapy of filariasis; effect of 1-diethyl-carbamyl-4-methylpiperazine hydrochloride against naturally acquired filarial infection in cotton rats and dogs." J. Lab. and Clin. Med. 32, 1314-1329.

Kobayachi, J., Takeo Bando, and Ishizacki. 1952. "Locomotion of Ascaris suilla et lumbricoides and the influence of anthelminthics upon them." Jap. J. Pharm. 1, 2, 130-143.

Lamson, P. D., Brown, H. W., Ward, C. B., and Robbins, B. N. 1930. "Hexylresorcinol in the treatment of hookworm disease." Proc. Soc. Exp. Biol. Med. 28, 1, 191-193.

Lamson, P. D., Brown, H. W., and Ward, C. B. 1935a. "Anthelminthic studies on alkylhydroxybenzenes, alkylpoly-hydroxybenzenes." J. Pharm. 53, 198-217.

Lamson, P. D., Brown, H. W., Stougton, K. W., Harwood, P. D., and Bass, A. K. 1935b. "Anthelminthic studies on alkylhydroxybenzenes. II. Ortho- and para-alkylphenols." J. Pharm. 53, 218-226.

Lamson, P. D., and Brown, H. W. 1935c. "Anthelminthic studies on alkylhydroxybenzenes, 6-n-alkyl-meta-cresols." J. Pharm. 53, 227-233.

Lamson, P. D., Brown, H. W., et al., 1935d. "Anthelminthic studies on alkylhydroxybenzenes, isomerism in poly-alkylphenols." J. Pharm. 53, 234-238.

Lamson, P. D., Brown, H. W., et al. 1935e. "Anthelminthic studies on alkylhydroxybenzenes, phenols with other than normal side chains." J. Pharm. 53, 239-249.

Lamson, P. D., and Ward, C. B. 1936. "Earthworms as test of drugs to be used in human intestinal helminth infesta-tions." Science 84, 2178, 293-294.

Lasarus, M., and Rogers, W. P. 1951. "The mode of action of phenothiazine as an anthelminthic. The uptake of S^{35}-labeled phenothiazine by the tissues of nematode parasites and their hosts." Australian J. Sci., Ser. B., Biol. Sci. 4, 2, 163-174.

Lawrence, J. H., Loomis, W. F., Tobias, C. A., and Turpin, F. H. 1946. "Preliminary observations on narcotic effect of xenon with review of values for solubilities of gases in water and oil." J. Physiol. 105, 197-204.

Le Dentu. 1949. Un ténifuge efficace et économique. La presse médicale. 32, 438.

Maplestone, P. A., and Chopra, R. N. 1934. "Effect of hexylresorcinol on cats." Indian J. Med. Res. 21, 219-251.

Maplestone, P. A., and Mukerji, A. K. 1931. "Carbon tetrachloride in treatment of taenia infections." Indian Med. Gazette 66, 567-570.

Niemirski, A. 1954. "Benzene in therapy of tapeworm infection." Polski tygodnik lek. 9, 211-213.

Oelkers, H. A. 1943. Pharmakologische Grundlagen der Behandlung von Wurmkrankheiten.

Oelkers, H. A., and Rathye, W. 1941. "Zur Wirkungsweise der Anthelmintica." Naunyn Schmiedebergs Arch. 198, 317-337.

Rebello, S., Gomes da Costa, S. F., and Rico J. Toscano. 1928. Sensibilité des cestodes á l'action de quelque anti-helminthiques." C. R. Soc. Biol. 96, 473-475.

Shideman, F. E., Kelly, A. K., and Adams, B. L. 1947. "Role of liver in detoxication of thiopental (pentothal) and two other thiobarbiturates." J. Pharm. 91, 331-339.

Spector, W. S. 1956. Handbook of Biological Data. Philadelphia-London.

Spector, W. S. 1957. Handbook of Toxicology. I. Philadelphia-London.

Todd, A. C., and Brown, K. G. 1952. "Critical tests with toluene for ascarids and bots in horses." Amer. J. Vet. Res. 13, 47, 198-200.

Wenzel, D. G., and Gibson, K. D. 1951. "Study of toxicity and anthelminthic activity of n-butylidene chloride." J. Pharmacy and Pharm. 3, 3, 169-176.

Whitlock, J. H. 1945. "Anthelminthic bioassay of simple saturated hydrocarbons." Cornell Veterinarian 35, 3, 214-220.

Wigand, R., and Warnecke, W. 1953. "Benzinum Petrolii (DAB) in der Therapie der Taeniasis (T. saginata)." Med. Klinik 48, 27, 964-965.

Wright, W. H. and Schaffer, J. M. 1932. "The comparative anthelminthic efficacy for ascarides and hookworms in the dog of halogenated hydrocarbons containing chlorine, bromine, and iodine." J. Parasitol. 18, 1, 44.

Wright, W. H., Schaffer, J. M., Bozicevich, J., and Underwood, P. C. 1937. "Critical anthelminthic tests of some primary monobromo hydrocarbons." Researches in Helminthology (edited by R. S. Shul'ts and Gnedin). Moscow, pp. 769-780.